SPECIAL OFFER

Simply Functional Medicine:

- Free One-On-One Consultation
  Spend 20-30 minutes working together to create a plan for getting you HEALTHY
- Everyone who applies for a consultation receives a gift

4 WAYS TO REGISTER

Mobile Text
Text to: 58885 your name and email with the keyword HEALTHY

Voice
Call 866-603-3995 PIN # 149963

Web
bonus.DrKrisSargent.com

QR Code

Table of Contents

Dedication 5

Acknowledgement 5

Part 1: The Rant 11

Chapter 1: **It's What They Know** 15

Chapter 2: **You Need a Team** 61

Chapter 3: **But It's So Yummy: CRAP** 73

Chapter 4: **C: Clean it Up** 87

Chapter 5: **R: Restore Function** 125

Chapter 6: **A: Action** 155

Chapter 7: **P: Personalized** 167

Conclusion 182

Congratulations! 183

Dedication

Dr. Kris Sargent ~

This book is dedicated to…

My family… My mom, Jean Sargent, the woman who has been my back-up taxi, kid-sitter, laundress, maid, prayer-warrior, loves me when I'm unlovable and never lets me down, 87-year-old Inspiration of amazing health! My dad, Phil Sargent, who is and has always been the model of non-judgmental attitude and solid faith, long-suffering ear to my seemingly endless tears for a few years, and master of puns. Dave Renard, my amazing partner who sees me in my crazy and loves me anyway and encourages it! Kallan and Cooper, my extraordinary children, who may have had less of me during this project, who were excited when I wasn't, and who have taught me more than I could ever imagine. I love you more than you will ever know.

Acknowledgement

This is my third attempt at writing a book. I have wanted to write one for about 10 years. I fully understand what it means to "get in your own way". I was firmly rooted in three things. First, what other people would think. What if I hurt someone's feelings or said something that would upset someone? Too bad, they have to manage their own emotions. Second, fear of people not liking my work or seeing the value. I wasn't sure I really had anything to say that hadn't already been said and I didn't want to let down my mentors. I vibrate at a frequency that will attract exactly who needs to be attracted, I have my own tribe. This led to the third fear. I did not see what God intended for me to be and how I was to "show up" in the world as the best version of myself! I found her! She's sassy, smart as heck, sexy and funny, but most of all passionately in love with Functional Medicine and all of the people she has helped and will help in the future.

Thank you to all my coaches: Vickie Austin, who helped me write my first marketing plan, delivered it 2 days before my daughter was born, and then helped me see how much I had accomplished 18 months later. Larry Markson, who could always see through my "Three enneagram" personality, who would call me out to be a better human and never stopped believing in me, and is available at a moment's notice, even 10 years later. Theresa Peterson Mendoza, my therapist and CBT guru, who saw me through some of my darkest days after my divorce while I was learning to be a parent to my amazing kids, and who saw my beautiful soul and strength even when I couldn't see it. Cindy Dove, who lovingly helped me wrap my head around a different practice model and a new vision for my life and of myself, some of that wasn't realized for 18 more months. Daryl Rivers, who finally asked the question enough times it sunk in, "When are you really going to LOVE yourself?" My ex-husband, David Anderson, who is a great dad, who I am blessed to call friend, and who also taught me lessons I never expected to learn.

And last but NOT least, Barry Schimmel, who helped me see the big picture of writing this book, then walked me through every detail (which I dislike immensely) until the book and online classes were complete, who kept prodding me to get out of my own way, get my mindset right and just get it done, and who ultimately reminded me how to dream big and accomplish my BHAG.

Big gratitude to Dr. Jeffrey Bland, for without his conception of the way medicine "should" be, i.e. Functional Medicine, I wouldn't have been able to help the thousands of patients up to now, and the millions I will help with this book and online classes.

Thank you to all of my patients, and the Hashimoto's Facebook group admins, Shawna, Heather, Des, Tracy and Dawn who ultimately allowed me to see my knowledge base for what it was - extensive! For all of you who suffer from Auto-immune disorders, Hashimoto's and others, there is hope!

Finally, (geez, I know, right?) I must thank my amazing partner, Dave Renard. Dave has been supportive of my quirkiness, poor planning and last-minuteness I call spontaneity, and basically allowing me to be "ME", and for giving me the inspiration and latitude to do what I do.

Dr Kris Sargent's Story

Dr Kris Sargent's interest in Functional Medicine was to solve some of her own health issues. She saw a chiropractor, on advice of her mom, for pain and blood sugar related fatigue at 19 years old. Her parents were always into healthy lifestyles. At this time, both of her parents at 85 and 87 are very healthy, independent, taking no medication, and live very active lives

As she went through chiropractic school and learned about nutrition and Functional Medicine her own PMS issues became overwhelming. She learned how to use nutrition and supplements to solve that issue and started telling all the women in her life, "you don't have to live with horrible periods". After having her children around 40 years old she suffered from postpartum depression, horrendous brain fog, thyroid and hormonal issues. Functional Medicine came to the rescue. Then, peri-menopause, menopause and a close brush with an auto-immune disorder brought on by stress, have been traversed successfully with Functional Medicine. She fully understands "I Feel Like CRAP!" Her personal experience created a keen sense for using a patient's health history, extensive laboratory testing and current symptoms to format unique solutions for patients.

Dr Kris Sargent is a cutting-edge expert in Functional Medicine. She creates personalized solutions for fatigue, weight loss, hormone issues, sleep, achiness and digestive problems. She graduated with degrees in Biology and Psychology from the University of Central Florida in 1988. Along with a B.S. in Human

Anatomy, she completed her Doctorate of Chiropractic degree at The University of Health Sciences in 1992. Over the years, Dr. Sargent has accumulated hundreds of hours of continuing education in Functional Medicine, Leadership and Personal Development, Certification in First Line Therapy, a post-doctoral Master's Degree in Advanced Clinical Practice.

Dr. Kris Sargent is a professional speaker, author, and physician/coach. With 26 years in practice, Dr. Sargent considers herself a clinical science geek and sleuth. And as a single mother, business owner and busy entrepreneur, she understands the importance of self-care for the strength and resilience necessary to positively move through the challenges of life.

Message to the World
You can Feel Fabulous! Feeling like CRAP is not acceptable. Being demeaned by Doctors is also not acceptable. You deserve to understand what is up with your health and find a reasonable solution involving primarily lifestyle changes.

Message intended for:

Women of all ages who are tired of Feeling Like CRAP. You're NOT crazy and you probably know more about your body and nutrition than your doctor. Trust your intuition.

Three things about me:

1) I get to the cause of the problem. I don't just cover it up with medications or cut it out. Essentially, I put a

plan in place for your body to heal itself. Your body already knows how to be healthy, given the right ingredients.
2) I specialize in women who have been everywhere and tried everything. I am the "last resort" Doctor.
3) I want everyone to know about the power of Functional Medicine

Give back attitude:

I consistently share my knowledge, making my protocols available to everyone with internet access, so the Medicine of the Future, Functional Medicine, can be used by all, NOW.

Purpose:

My purpose is to create a Revolution in Medicine by bring the future of Medicine to everyone, now, in a Do It Yourself format, so more people will have access to this real "HEALTH-Care", and not rely solely on the current "SICK-care" model.

Part 1: The Rant

"My doctor doesn't listen to me."

"My doctor ignores my symptoms and says my labs are normal."

"I spent a lot of time and gathered research and was demeaned and demoralized for thinking it was true."

I asked for some different labs and my doctor won't run them because the insurance won't cover them; or he just refused, or says they aren't necessary, or tells me to stay off the internet, or that the side effects are so rare that I am probably not experiencing them."

"My doctor said what I eat doesn't influence my digestion," (one of my personal favorites), my doctor says, "nutrition doesn't have any effect on my acne, autoimmune disorder... (insert any disease process)".

"I played by the rules, went to all the HMO doctors I was supposed to, spent $1000's of dollars on copays and things that weren't covered, and I still don't have any answers, except a handful of prescriptions and I have all of the side effects possible, and all my doctors think I'm crazy."

"I am beginning to think I AM crazy, because my doctors have told me nothing is wrong, but I still feel like crap!"

This is just a handful of the complaints I hear on a daily basis from patients about the typical medical doctors and specialists experiences. Some highly trained physicians, at teaching hospitals, and still these women (most of my patient base is comprised of women), are still NOT getting any answers. This is NOT okay!

Before I continue, I want to say something VERY IMPORTANT! I am NOT opposed to ALL of the traditional healthcare and insurance system in America. Frankly, if I am having a heart attack, or I need my acute appendix removed, or I am in a severe accident, I want our doctors to do what they do best - act appropriately in an acute, potentially life-threatening situation. Our doctors excel in these situations, you cannot get any better. I was very grateful for the doctors who diagnosed my pneumonia when I was pregnant with Cooper, my son. I was also grateful of the admittance to the hospital and for the three days of IV antibiotics for the pneumonia consuming both of my lungs. Yes, I totally understand the need, time and place.

I am writing this book to help explain why so many of us are not getting the answers we deserve. I am writing this book to help explain why you are not getting the answers you deserve. I am also writing this to explain why Americans, specifically, are so unhealthy, overweight and obese. 70% overweight and obese to be exact! Yes, we are "the most in debt, obese, addicted, and medicated adult cohort in US history" to quote one of my favorite authors, Brene Brown. Lastly, I am writing this book to spark a change in your soul, so that you can brighten your world every day.

This is not okay...

It's not! And I'm going to bat for you. It's not okay to pay money into a system that doesn't have the philosophy to actually help people until they are SO sick, that their body is completely worn out from trying to compensate for poor habits. It's not okay that the medical schools do not teach nutrition to our doctors.

It's not okay for our doctors, MD's DO's and DC's to be dismissive and demeaning to patients, who may actually have knowledge their doctor cannot possibly have time to learn.

It's also not okay for doctors to make recommendations regarding nutrition since they have not been trained in nutrition. If I made recommendations about prescription meds, I lose my license. How is it that they can basically say anything to a patient and get away with it? And most patients do not even question them. I am very passionate about this, if you couldn't tell.

I really don't like to think that what I offer is "Alternative". I offer simple, common sense solutions that have to do with everyday life. Solutions that have to do with what we eat and drink, how we move, sleep, think and feel.

When did eating vegetables, fruit and lean proteins become alternative medicine? This is ludicrous!

Although I have been in this mind set since I was nineteen years old, I am still learning every day! My patients alert me to new things all the time. There are hundreds of them and only one of me. Of course, they have more eyes and ears than I could ever have on the internet. I learn new things all the time. I'm just not so short sighted or egotistical to believe I learned everything in chiropractic school.

Why haven't the traditional doctors and specialists in this country done the same? I can't answer for them. What I do know is there are other answers to getting to health! Scripts and scalpels may or may not be involved!

Above all, you <u>need</u> to know, NO, you are not crazy!

Chapter 1: It's What They Know

Script or scalpel?

At eight years old, I will never forget the horrible experience I had with a medical doctor. My mom had taken me in to our family physician because I was sick, again, with strep throat. Although mom had been a chiropractic patient since her early 20's, she took us kids to the "regular" doctor. On this particular visit, mind you, I went in for a sore throat, the doctor looked at me and said, "you are going to be 300 pounds by the time you're 19 if you keep gaining weight." Not exactly a thing you tell an 8-year-old, who danced 4 days a week and swam almost every day. And whose mom cooked homemade, real food. He gave me no instructions on how to stop gaining or how to lose weight. He was demeaning. I hated going to the doctor after that, and feigned being well, even when I was sick, so I wouldn't have to go again. A doctor is supposed to be compassionate and know how to "first do no harm".

Did that one event change the trajectory of my life? Yes, it certainly was instrumental. Did I struggle with my weight and body image? You bet! That incident combined with several other life factors. My mom and sister were naturally thin. I was more muscular. I had a dance teacher than forced weight loss before the recital every year. We moved around a lot when I was growing up so, I didn't have an established group of friends. I assumed kids didn't like me because I was "fat".

As I matured I went on to face-down many of those inaccurate self-limiting beliefs. It is a journey. Writing this book, is the culmination of finding my true inner voice and listening to it. That voice helped me see my passion for creating a healthier America. I am a true patriot at heart.

My personal awareness allowed me to see so many women wrangling with the same issues I battled with without a place to turn. They try so many things and fail. They actually lose trust in themselves and they lose hope. Having a family doctor that is not helping you is not okay. They are supposed to be on your side. I am on your side. That it part of what drove me to be a physician in the first place. Yes, a chiropractic physician, because that profession aligned with my personal health philosophy and value system.

When I was in college in the 1980's, I decided on a "pre-med" track. I ended up with degrees in Biology and Psychology. I was, ironically, studying to be a medical doctor. I remembered the experiences I had as a kid and wanted to be a different kind of doctor. One that would listen and be kind to patients. One day, after complaining of neck and shoulder pain, my mom said I should see her chiropractor. I had a history of two car accidents and I had danced, ballet, for 15 years, so plenty of neck strain over time. I had never had any treatment except the standard medical care of some muscle relaxers and aspirin. So, as any good daughter would at 19 years old, I rolled my eyes and sighed, and promptly made an appointment. That visit changed my life.

I learned about the nervous system and its role in our body. I learned that getting a chiropractic adjustment could change the nervous system and therefore, change the way my body functioned. It all made sense to me. The chiropractor also gave me some ideas about carrying my books, what to eat for better energy, encouraged me to keep dancing and stretching, he asked me about sleep and hydration. Then, he went on to give me a plan to help my neck and shoulders. This is now known as lifestyle medicine. Chiropractors have been practicing this way for way over 100 years. This was at a time when the "lifestyle medicine" concept was not a thing, and there was not an internet!

That chiropractor used simple solutions like changing what I was eating, drinking, how I was moving, sleeping, thinking and feeling to help me heal. His little black bag was clearly full of more tools than my medical doctor. Chiropractic aligned with my personal health philosophy and my value system. It was decided, I was going to be a chiropractor. Little did I know the uphill battle that awaited me. My dad, my college advisor, friends, all questioned why I didn't want to become a "real" doctor and did I know they weren't even licensed? The licensure part wasn't true, as were many other lies people believed, then and still do, about chiropractors and chiropractic.

At one point, I was going for a prestigious position on campus as part of an elite group of students known as the President's Leadership Council. We would represent the University when visitors were on campus. There was an application process and an interview. The interview included faculty, Dean's and my advisor. I actually had to defend my choice to become a chiropractor during that interview! It was the first time I really felt like an outcast in the medical world, but not the last time I had to defend my choice.

After almost 10 years of school and 25 years in practice, I am still faced with statements like, "Oh, what is a chiropractor doing in a Hashimoto's Facebook group when medical doctors don't even understand the thyroid?", or the downward gaze and "OOH" when I tell people I am a chiropractor and people have called me a fraud, a quack and a snake oil salesman. (Um, I'm a girl, not a man.) Painful? Yes. I wouldn't be honest if I said it didn't bother me. For years, I would let those statements get under my skin and erode my confidence and self-worth. By 2007 my life trajectory changed. I was ready to quit practice, it was too overwhelming with 2 kids, a husband, practice, perfectionism effecting every corner of my life. My self-esteem was in the toilet. I had really hit a low. Most people had no idea what was happening on the inside. Even my husband didn't fully understand. How could he? I didn't even understand. On the outside, everything looked perfect, right? Two kids, a girl and a boy, beautiful home, great husband, by most accounts a successful practice of 15 years and I was on a path to implosion.

The only thing that kept me going at that time was my faith. I will discuss this more, suffice it to say, God's timing is impeccable. Through a colleague of mine I was re-introduced to the principles of success. I was reminded of the essential truths of the Bible and Napoleon Hill. I had several mentors over the last few years that landed me in a very different place, mentally, spiritually, emotionally and physically.

Just so you know, that transformation did not happen in a flash or with some magic pill. It was as painful as the way I had been living. It became a matter of what was worse, my current reality or the pain of real change.

That's what this book is about. It's about a shift, not only mindset, but how you approach your health habits and how you can heal much of your life with small habit changes over time. I no longer take personal offense. Oh, it still stings a little, but I am able to see it as an opportunity to explore a person's value system. Now, I take it as an opportunity to ask questions, and educate. People can't know what they don't know, ignorance about chiropractic and medical alternatives is still abundant.

Hey, you may have had a positive, negative or no experience whatsoever with chiropractic or chiropractors. If your experience was positive - awesome, and welcome! If you have no experience - awesome, and welcome! If you have had a negative experience, all I ask is for a second chance. There are bad people and experiences in every profession. Those experiences do not have to define your relationship with them forever. So awesome, and welcome!

The internet has made a difference. People are starting to see there are alternatives for healing or even "curing" disease. We were always taught to use the word "cure" very carefully. The body has an odd way of relapsing. But, I can tell you I have seen miracle after miracle, from chiropractic adjustments and combined lifestyle changes for tens of thousands of patients.

In many respects, medical education is nothing like chiropractic education. Most medical schools do not teach the recommended 25 hours nutrition, or alternatives like herbs, vitamins, stress management skills, water consumption guidelines, exercise plans, sleep hygiene, acupuncture, energy medicine, weight loss strategies or health-related modalities.

They are taught system pathology. Pathology is the study of diseases at the tissue and cellular level. They belief that the body is continually getting old, and there is not much that can be done. Regardless of the literature screaming otherwise, typical MD's sneer at the connection of lifestyle to health and disease. The philosophy doesn't really encompass the fact that the body can actually heal itself. Which, for many of us, the idea that all the systems are connected, is just common sense. Interestingly, chiropractic schools do have to teach about all of the "ologies"…. Gynecology, pulmonology, urology, gastroenterology, otolaryngology, neurology, orthopedics, pathology as well, you get the picture. Look up the catalog for National University of Health Sciences, one of the most academically based chiropractic schools in the country, and my AlmaMater. Chiropractic schools are required to teach clinical diagnosis of the entire body. We are required to learn pharmacology, prescription drugs and how they work in the body, even though in most states we do not have the license to prescribe. We still must learn it. Most medical schools do not even teach basic nutrition! Seriously? I know, right!?

Traditional Medicine is only concerned with the actual disease of a body part. That's why there are so many of the "-ologies". Each is a subset of organs of the body with a specialist for everyone. And even though the organ systems talk to each other through a dizzying array of cellular chemistry, the specialists rarely speak to each other. The patient is left to communicate between highly trained specialists. They believe that disease is inherent in the person, it comes from your genetics. Once you have it, there is very little you can do to heal yourself. You will just have to live with the cards that you were dealt. They are not trained to look for WHY or WHAT caused the issue in the first place. They are not trained to look at where the physiology is breaking down, or what the cause of the breakdown could be.

For example, if you have a flat tire, there could be several causes. You could have a nail in it, or it just wore out and won't hold air, or you totally trashed the tire by running over a curb or down a pot-hole filled road. OR it might just need air. So, instead of looking for the cause - the typical traditional doctor approach is to just change the whole tire or try to patch it together with some new-fangled rubber-like substance that will act like rubber.

They are trained to monitor labs and your symptoms. As long as both are fine, in the range of the general population, you must be fine. We will discuss lab values later in the book. Optimal health lab values and standard lab ranges are very different and are not even used the same way. If you come in with symptoms they do NOT have a pill for, frankly, they have no idea what to do for you. Their tool bag is small. It only contains a Script and a Scalpel.

Yes, they will test what is covered by your insurance company or what the latest study told them was minimally necessary. They are not trained to look any further. The crazy thing is, we were all taught the same physiology. When the body becomes ill, it produces a symptom to tell you that something is wrong. It may be a disruption at the cellular level, like insulin resistance, type 2 diabetes, or it may be a disruption at the organ level like gallstones. In any case, instead of fixing the dysfunction, or what caused the dysfunction, they fix the symptom.

Let's look at a simplified version of blood pressure. Blood pressure increases and decreases through the day depending on the demands of the body. When you are going up a flight of stairs, you want more blood pressure to force the oxygenated blood to your muscles, so you can climb the stairs. Our blood pressure can also increase to different stresses such as increased weight or dehydration. Instead of really addressing the weight issue, except in a passing comment like "you need to drop some weight", you are handed a script and told to keep a log of your blood pressure. There is not even a mention of the water or hydration as a key factor in keeping blood pressure normal, or that a lack of magnesium could also cause some of the problem. Also, did you know that your blood pressure is supposed to rise and fall depending on where your body may need oxygen and nutrients at any given moment.

Because the philosophy is one of "get rid of symptoms and the patient is fine" traditional doctors have no need to look further. When you return with similar or worse symptoms they will increase your medication, give you a second one or the newest one that is stronger, or (with snarkiness intended) they give you the one their drug rep just dropped off a couple days prior. You may not want to know that part, or you may already know the way Pharma works.

The crazy thing about many blood pressure medications is they slow down the whole body. The side effects are drowsiness, sexual dysfunction, foggy brain, not exactly a recipe for getting healthy. Diabetes, is also a known side effect of some of these medications. So, now you are on two blood pressure medications and your blood sugar and cholesterol come back elevated on a lab test and BOOM! You are on two more meds to lower the sugar and cholesterol; the root problem still has not been addressed. Even if the person "feels fine", there are underlying problems still lurking. Your doctor may have even gone so far as to tell you to find a weight loss plan or erroneously told you to quit eating so much fat in your diet. But, more commonly, your doctor handed you a script. These medications are known as "Lifestyle Drugs" and comprise eight of the top ten medications prescribed in the US.

So, hang with me for a minute. Have you ever known someone who you had seen just a few days before, then you heard they had a heart attack or even died? Maybe this person was even "healthy". According to that person, they felt "great". I don't know about you, I have often wondered, then why did they suddenly have a heart attack? Feeling good and being symptom free is not synonymous with HEALTH. Here's the truth, 50% of people who have heart attacks have normal cholesterol.

Do you think there is something else going on? Do you think, just maybe, there is another way to look at health instead of masking symptoms and waiting for diseases to take over?

Another analogy, what if your "Check Engine" light came on in your car? You decided it was an annoying light, so you looked under the hood for the wire to the light and cut the wire or you just stuck some duct tape over the dashboard light. AHHH, relief, no more annoying light! But, how long do you think you will be able to ignore the problem before some other annoying light comes on or the entire engine just seizes up? Isn't there still an engine problem? What is the root of that light turning on in the first place?

Is there still an underlying health issue?

This is how the traditional medical profession looks at your body's symptoms, like the check engine light blazing. They can medicate your symptoms into oblivion, but the root cause of the illness is ignored. Yet, the disease process is still ongoing.

The worst part is the medical profession is inadequately trained in lifestyle medicine like nutrition. There is research back to 1990 and as recent as 2016 stating the inadequacy of nutrition training. They acknowledge the problem, but have not been able to change it. The graduate medical educators know there is a huge problem. This is not just here in the US, but also Canada, and less in Europe.

So, the offhanded comment about losing weight is really all they may know about really regaining your health. Even when I was 8 years old, and was told to lose weight, no actual solution was given at the time. The fact that I had recurring strep throat was also not addressed. I was demeaned for being fat, given more antibiotics and sent home. Some doctors take the snide approach and demean their patients by saying things like, "calories in, calories out" when weight loss and lifestyle is much more complicated that just calories. I have heard it all.

What is even more insidious is the demeaning attitude of traditional medical doctors and the medical profession as a whole, towards lifestyle medicine. For a centuries, chiropractors and naturopaths, have been discredited because we are not "real" doctors because we cannot prescribe drugs, and that our education is inadequate. Yet when you look into the hours these "alternative" professions spend learning about pharmaceuticals, plus nutrition, I think you will agree, it is the medical profession that is now undereducated in the ills of this country.

If the top drugs are being prescribed because of lifestyle issues, and the medical profession isn't trained in lifestyle medicine, how is it that the chiropractic and naturopathic professions are the inadequately trained? How is it that these professions are still considered "not real doctors"? They can hide behind the money of the insurance and pharmaceutical companies who support their philosophy. They do not have the new tools of Lifestyle medicine. I feel sorry for them, they only have a Script and a Scalpel.

Philosophy, Pharma and Protection

Boring, right? Not this time. Let's take a deeper dive into the traditional medical philosophy in this country. The philosophy or thought process that runs through the minds of the typical medical doctor is actually fascinating and sad. For the record, I know many doctors who have shifted their thinking to one extent or another. I also know some wonderful traditional doctors who treat their patients with love and dignity. I commend and revere each of these hard-working loving docs. I will also reiterate the need for their training in acute situations. I definitely want one on my side if I have an acute event in my life! They are the best trained physicians in the world for those moments.

The majority of traditional doctors in America have many constraints created by several forces. Some of those forces are out of the direct control of the doctor and are part of our system. I am sure I will say some things that will irritate some of you. Please hear me out. Who pays for care is irrelevant when the basic foundation of the medical educational system is broken. The medical education system has nothing to do with keeping people healthy. It is concerned with disease management. It only looks for and treats symptoms and end stage diseases. The system is designed to only pay for illness. It is not set up to keep people healthy in the first place. Please do not expect your insurance company to keep you healthy.

Let's look at your home owner's insurance or your car insurance. Does your auto insurance pay for oil changes or new tires? When was the last time your home owner's insurance paid for new windows or to paint the exterior of your home? Health insurance isn't designed to take care of your body. It is designed to take care of you when something happens. Just like when you get into an auto accident or a tornado rips off your roof. Does your health insurance pay for your gym membership? Your bottled water? Your vegetables and fruit? I am not against insurance, it's just NOT an entitlement policy. I am not against using pharmaceuticals to keep people comfortable who are in need, have infections, pain, and/or cancer. But, there is another side. And humans need both.

I am against the proliferation of scripts that are used to treat people who refuse to change or take on a small shift in how they are treating their body or pull themselves up by the bootstraps and change their lifestyle when the donuts and fast food they are consuming, are starting a disease process.

The American relationship with food is completely dysfunctional. We use food for everything except actually nourishing our bodies. I am also not opposed to eating junk food occasionally. Food is fuel not fun...at least not fun everyday...Geez, I love popcorn and key lime pie. Dr Andersen, of Medifast/Optavia, teaches to Stop... Challenge... Choose. Stop and pay attention to what you are doing when you are about to grab for some unhealthy. What is the challenge in front of you? Why is it so attractive and what are the options? Then, make a choice. I generally choose to eat popcorn once or twice a month now. I eat key lime pie on my birthday. I use my weight as data to guide me through treating myself. We will talk about these and other strategies for creating a healthier lifestyle later in the book.

It's not a mystery that processed and fast, causes poisoned and fat.

70% of the American population, YES 70%, of Americans are obese and overweight. This is not by accident and there is NOT a drug to date that can cure fat. Yes, there, I said it. It's literally the elephant in the room. Yes, I just said that too! Get sense of humor, laughter IS medicine. It's been shown to add years to your life. Basic principles of what you eat and drink, how you move, sleep, think and feel create health or disease for the majority of us.

To clarify, I am not opposed to all medication. Mental illness is real. There are life-saving drugs and cancer fighting miracles. I am not so naive to think that zero medications should be used.

When we are discussing lifestyle drugs, I prefer to keep someone on medications as they shift and heal. For example, keeping someone on blood pressure medication while they lose weight and exercise. I am not talking about everyone having a perfect body, just get your weight into a relatively healthy range and exercise at least 3 hours a week, 30 minutes a day, 6 days a week. We can all find 30 minutes a day.

I also heartily believe that the body has tremendous ability to heal itself given the right ingredients and environment.

Health is 70-90% environment (what our body is exposed to - eat, drink, move, sleep, think and feel) plus 10-30% genetics. Your health is only partially determined by your genetics! Your DO NOT have to "Live with it" ... whatever chronic issue you have, you have the power to change it

We have the coolest defense and repair system programmed into our body. It's like having a car that will take itself to the repair shop for routine maintenance. How cool is that?!!

When we sleep and eat healthy food our maintenance centers can work properly. Our maintenance centers involve the brain and nervous system and our immune system. These systems in our body were created to defend us from mental and emotional stress, poor food and drink choices, and invaders, bacteria, fungi/yeast and viruses, let's refer to these as our personal super heroes.

It starts in what I call our Automatic Nervous System, officially known as the autonomic nervous system. It senses the stressor and talks to our immune system through chemical messengers. Part of the immune system rushes in and repairs cells, organs and tissues, all by itself, it knows what to do and how to do it. Our bodies are amazing. We don't even have to think about it. So, I do not believe we are destined to be sick, once we have a "disease". Our bodies are always trying to heal. It's what we do when we rest - we repair. When we sleep, our body goes to work to fix broken parts and clean up the mess we make during the day.

I have seen too many people heal, or go into remission from any number of diseases, from diabetes and heart disease to cancer and auto-immune disorders. Too many to just be a coincidence. I have not performed a double blind, placebo-controlled trial, I have lived thousands of stories with thousands of people over 25 years. I do, however, have thousands of N=1, personal stories. I could seriously rant right now, but will hold back until later in the chapter.

Bottom Line...the body IS designed to heal itself. How well will your body heal when all it has been fed is from the junk yard? When we feed the body what it needs, it can create healing chemistry, and our body will heal.

Philosophy, Genetics, Genomics

I began to describe the way medical doctors think about your body and diseases. I believe it deserves a little more explanation. Since we are all taught the same physiology or the way the body functions, something must happen when people enter medical school that changes the perception of basic human physiology.

Our perception is our reality. How we look at any situation or fact is seen through our own set of lenses. Those lenses have been colored by many things such as stuff we saw our parents do, what we experienced and learned as kids, how we were taught, what part of the world and culture we were raised in, and our own experiences with our health as we matured. You get the idea. Our beliefs about our health and our ability to change our health were shaped just like all of our beliefs about the world in general. A belief system that surrounds health is rarely discussed. We talk about religion, politics and sex, but health isn't exactly as sexy as that, although once entered, you will find it just as hotly debated as any of the taboo topics.

I grew up in a fairly conservative home, with conservative values. I grew up Christian, republican, Episcopalian. That may or may not BE who I am today, because I have looked long and hard at my own beliefs and have made my own decisions.

I have become hyper-aware of my thought processes and what underlying belief systems shape my day to day lifestyle choices. I also grew up with a mom who had always seen a chiropractor, who took vitamins, and made all our food from scratch. My dad, on the other hand, was fairly medical in his health model. Although, he took vitamins, ate healthy because of my mom, and he softened as I showed him research article after research article about chiropractic care and lifestyle medicine, in general.

My mom is a healthy almost 87 at the time I am writing this, and my dad just celebrated a healthy 85th birthday. Neither take medication. Age and aging are just numbers, and do NOT have to be horrible or painful. What our society thinks as aging at 30, 40 or 50 doesn't have to be! You do not have to have a slow, steady decline in health from age 35 to 70 and then die a miserable death. You can be a healthy, vibrant productive citizen until you are 100 years old or more, and then just die without much suffering.

Poor aging is usually about neglect. Again, I know there are many people that have accidents, infections, things happen to us in life that we don't always intend, and we can still live long lives. I repeat, poor aging is generally about neglect. Neglecting to actually "get around to it". Get around to choosing healthy, getting around to exercise…you get the picture. Is it time for you to get around to it?

The key to the philosophical differences is genetics. Here is a little science lesson from seventh grade. We all probably learned about Mendel and his peas. Mendelian genetics basically says that our DNA, which is housed deep in the nucleus of our cell, programs our body and physiology, is what it is…it is not capable of change so, we are just a product of our genes. This is known as our genotype. Our hair color, how tall we are, the shape of our nose and our body, the diseases we get, all genetically pre-programmed.

However, back in 1990, The Human Genome project began to sequence our DNA. "That is awesome Dr Kris", you are thinking, "YAAWWNN… what the heck is that and what a geek!!" (insert appropriate eye roll emoji) Yes, I am a geek and I love genetics. Here's what you need to know. Since that time, 1990, we have discovered that our genetic expression, our phenotypes, are not pre-programmed. There are some rare exceptions of course! We still may have a tendency toward a certain disease, however, our genetics only play a 10-30% role in actually getting that disease. YES! Really! So, what we were born with doesn't totally determine our health.

Just because you mom, dad, aunt, your entire family had a certain disease, doesn't necessarily mean you will get that same disease. Two things are in play here. First, how we treat our DNA will be, to a greater extent, the path of our health. This is our lifestyle. Only 10-30% of our health outcomes as we age have to do with genetics. And in case you suck at math, that leaves 70-90% in YOUR control. Second, the reasons diseases still appear to run in families are the deeply engrained family traditions and lifestyles that we have learned from our parents, the town or neighborhood we grew up in and our friends.

Let me say this another way. We learned to eat, drink, move, sleep, think and feel from our family. How much of what we have learned is negatively influencing our genetics?

When I was little we made tons of sweets and carbohydrate laden dishes around the Christmas holidays. My mom made two or three pies for Thanksgiving and lots of Christmas cookies. She also made everything from scratch. We had fresh meats and vegetables and very little processed foods. She made real mac-n-cheese, not from a box. She also taught me how to cook. I am very fortunate.

As I am now teaching my children to cook, I have been aware that we don't eat all the sweets she used to make, and I am refining what I am making for my family, because I am very aware of the risk of diabetes that runs in my family. The foods that I grew up eating were generally healthy, and my health is a result of those food choices that were instilled by my family. And, the genetic risk for diabetes? Well, because I have treated my genetics gently and not overtaxed them, I do not have the same issues as other family members.

Genetics is NOT a predetermined outcome. It is one you can control. So, if your family of origin and the society you grew up in is not healthy, then you will have those tendencies. You grew up in a culture that may have been healthy, or maybe not so much.

It may look like it's genetic, but our environment can have up to a 90% effect on how our genes are turned on or off.

I'll say it again and in yet another way: Health is 70-90% environment (what our body is exposed to - eat, drink, move, sleep, think and feel) plus 10-30% genetics. Your health is only partially determined by your genetics! Your DO NOT have to "Live with it". Whatever chronic issue you have, you have the power to change it.

The other piece of genetics that must not be ignored are individual traits that pop up in the populations. 23 and Me is a company that will give you a read of all your genes. You can learn about your specific genetic code. With some homework and a genetic specialist, you can learn about your genetic tendencies and what makes your body tick. You can then adjust your lifestyle, food intake, vitamin intake, and exercise to maximize your genetic potential. You may be able to avoid family diseases all together. I also offer a couple of genetic tests that will specifically identify what macros will work best for you. See my website, DrKrisSargent.com.

Some of these individual characteristics may leave your body deficient in certain vitamins because you don't process or absorb them well. This can lead to symptoms that might be mistaken for depression, anxiety, fatigue, hormone imbalances, irritable bowel syndrome and autoimmune disorders. The medical doctors aren't trained to look for those deficiencies or even blow them off if they are found, and you may be given a prescription for the symptoms. Just know, even though you may feel better, and in some cases, this is necessary, but the root of the issue has not been addressed. These prescriptions do not create the environment for your body to heal.

Here is the real crux of the problem. Traditional Medical doctors, as I said earlier, do not take classes in clinical nutrition! So, they do not know how to diagnose, or understand how all of the nutrition fits into our defense and repair system.

I am about to geek out on you, just FYI. They are not taught that your DNA needs a system called methylation to protect itself and to convert B-complex vitamins, including folate and B-12 into usable forms, to clear heart disease causing homocysteine from your body. They also don't generally know that a specific gene shift, called a single nucleotide polymorphism or SNP (pronounced "snip"), known as the MTHFR gene, can play a profound role in someone's health. This is just one example. I have seen hundreds of missed iron and B-12 deficiency anemias, people walking around with Vitamin D levels of 6 (should be 50-80 when healthy), missed thyroid issues and thousands of patients with other deficiencies.

The lack of knowledge or acceptance of this knowledge has led to countless doctor visits for what I call "I Feel Like CRAP Syndrome". YES! The impetus for the book title! CRAP lifestyle is the problem, it is also the symptom AND it is also going to be the solution! These patients feel terrible and are often dismissed or handed an antidepressant. Even if the doctor tests these patients for B-12 and folate deficiencies, they will likely not find them with the current lab tests.

These vitamins are water soluble. So, if you consume anything with these vitamins, it will show up in your blood, but the question then becomes is my body able to use these vitamins, and that depends on the genetics. This is a functional issue. The B-12 may be in your blood, but it needs to get into your bone marrow, and into your cells to actually do its job.

Because of genetics, you might not be able to transform the B-12 or folate into the correct and usable form. Your body may need some extra co-factors to make this happen. The traditional doctor has never been trained to look at MCV, as part of a normal CBC and homocysteine or methylmalonate, to determine what is actually happening in the body with the B-12 and folate. Unfortunately, the doctor assumes nothing is wrong and the patient is made to feel demeaned or dismissed, when they are scared and vulnerable, intuitively know something else is going on.

The upside for me was that I was in college and chiropractic school at this time. I was exposed to, at that time, the latest research, and I found mentors like Dr Jeffery Bland, the founder and father of Functional Medicine. Dr Bland has a long list of credentials, and is a pre-eminent biochemist who studied with Linus Pauling, the Father of Vitamin C. He is a visionary and wrote a book about how nutrition changes our genetic expression in 1999. Genetic Nutritioneering. YES! 1999! I poured through that book and have known for almost 30 years that what we eat determines our health outcomes more than our genetics. Thank you Dr Bland!

So, back to the medical side of this equation. By now you must be wondering how is this possible? How can our medical profession be so far behind in knowledge about health? They are well trained in how our body creates disease, but have no clue how to keep the body healthy. The medical profession has always been very slow to accept new ideas.

Joseph Lister, who developed the first antiseptic surgical methods, published his findings in a journal in 1867, but were not widely used until 1879! Seriously, he showed doctors how to kill less people on the operating table by hand washing and providing more sterile instruments and it took 12 years for the British medical community to decide this was a good idea. Most experts believe the medical profession can take up to 50 years to accept new information. YES! 50 years!

In this age of information and the rapidity with which information is spread and research is published, our traditional medical community is at least 50 years behind the times! That coupled with the next two topics, Pharma and Protection, creates a medical community who is out of touch with the health issues of mainstream Americans. You can know more than your doctor about nutrition and other subjects because you have taken the time to do the research.

Their perceptions are clouded by antiquated ideas about nutrition and lifestyle. The knowledge Dr Bland and the geneticists of the 1990's is just now being unearthed in the medical community, it's almost 40 years later and is still not widely accepted as truth, at all. (Insert large eye-roll and exasperated sigh, where is my emoji?)

As an aside, I took a certification course in 2002 called Genomics. An obscure lab, at the time, offered bits and pieces of what "23 and Me" does every day. The genetic tests were cumbersome and expensive. But, since 2002, we have had the ability to look at MTHFR, APO-A, APO-E and other SNP's that are greatly effected by what we eat, our lifestyle choices, and the type of supplements we need. It's <u>not</u> important for you to understand all the genetics here, suffice it to say, we have known for a long time that genes are influenced by what we eat, drink, how we move, how we sleep, our attitudes, thoughts and feelings. Therefore, YOU can control up to 90% of your health! This is now at your fingertips and not expensive. You buy food! You may need to change the type of food you buy.

A quick aside about the notion that eating healthy is expensive. When you start to shift your lifestyle, you will also shift what you spend your money on! Buying the junk, stopping at Starbucks or Dunkin' will not be part of your routine. Figure out your real food budget. Include all those little stops. Track it for a week. Also, track all your medication copays. When you start to eat healthy, you will be shifting from a $3 bag of Dorito's to a $3 bag of carrots. Both orange and crunchy. One promotes disease, one prevents disease. It's YOUR choice.

The solution is simple, not always easy. At the very least, the traditional medical profession as a whole needs to acknowledge they don't know everything. They need to admit that professing a clean lifestyle eating real food, lean protein fruits and vegetables is not going to hurt anyone.

And YES! Society plays a role. The majority expect their doctor to know everything. Patients should expect their doctor to have their best interest wrapped up in their recommendation. AND, patients want the quick fix, so they can get on their life. Doing the work of shifting habits that may have been engrained as a kid is not easy. However, it may save your life.

It seems crazy to think that simple instructions such as "eat real food" is considered alternative and controversial!?? Please understand, these statements can literally get your doctor in trouble. The insurance companies watch the types and numbers of prescription each doctor prescribes. If a Doctor chooses to start prescribing less and educating more, she can be reprimanded and possibly lose her license! It's crazy making!

Ideally, docs need to refer patients to the appropriate chiropractor or naturopath. A simple referral is all it would take to change the lives of millions of patients doomed to end up on the Script merry-go-round.

Another change that needs to happen is medical students need to take clinical nutrition for at least a year. They need to relearn laboratory diagnosis, to look at the physiology and systems biology. They can still prescribe medications, AND educate the patient choose to a lifestyle change first. The medical doctor doesn't have to practice lifestyle medicine, they will at least have knowledge of both sides, they can refer the patient, not dismiss and demean them. Doctors can choose how they want to practice and patients will have the choice of how they want to treat their body.

Um, how does that harm anyone?

The basic understanding that all systems work together, not separately in a vacuum, is necessary to bring medical education up to date with the current understanding of health and disease. In addition to medical education understanding the value of Lifestyle Medicine or Functional Nutrition or Functional Medicine, the diagnostic labs need to get on board with appropriate reference ranges for healthy people.

Do you know that the American Board of Clinical Endocrinologists approved a change for TSH, thyroid stimulating hormone, in 2002!! And most labs still have the old numbers on their reference ranges! This is crazy.

Hopefully, you are beginning to understand the missing components of our current system. The current system is broken. Who pays for care is irrelevant when the basic foundation of the medical educational system is broken. Health is not part of their philosophy. They are educated in the disease model and do not really acknowledge the body can heal itself.

Pharma

Yes, the pharmaceutical industry has played a role in the medical philosophy and our current medical system, at least here in the United States. With the invention of antibiotics in the 1930's, the pharmaceutical industry has played a pivotal role in our health. It has produced some amazing miracles and just as many catastrophes along the way. Neither of which I am going to go into too much as it is not the purpose of this book.

When antibiotics were introduced, it was easy to see the correlation. Bacteria invade the body, one bug, and causes and infection. There is a substance, called an antibiotic, one drug, which will kill the bug, and the body can heal. One bug, one drug. One pill for one ill. (Thank you, Dr Bland)

In 1907, we were alerted to the fact that probiotics in the intestine effected our health, thank you Elie Metchnikoff. His work was quoted in some of the original antibiotic research, in the 1930's. It was known that probiotics should always be taken with antibiotics! And again, 80 years later, medical doctors are just now accepting this fact.

HELLO! 80 years later!

The problem with the one bug, one drug theory is that Pharma isn't just treating infections anymore. The top drugs are known as "Lifestyle drugs". This means the diseases that are being treated by these drugs are because of our "Lifestyles". 70% of Americans are overweight and obese because the typical American lifestyle is the Standard American Diet (SAD) or aka Modern Urban Diet (MUD). And you wonder why you feel like CRAP after eating SAD MUD??

Drinking plenty caffeine and some alcohol, leading a generally sedentary life complaining of insomnia, Americans medicate. Most are really frustrated with the conflicting news of what to eat through our mainstream media outlets. They are left with a somewhat hopeless sense of ever being able to change any of those habits. They have tried and failed so many times. Many have given up altogether because they have lacked the proper support and direction. Habits are hard to change. So is sticking in the current reality of a broken healthcare system, where 70% of the patients are sick and getting sicker. What is wrong with this picture - this is NOT HEALTH care; it is SICK care.

High blood sugar, high blood pressure, and high cholesterol lowering drugs top the list, along with a handful of antidepressants and anti-anxiety drugs. Again, please do not think these medications aren't necessary in some cases. But, these drugs come with tons of side effects, that are sometimes longer than the commercials for the drug. AND, the drug is only treating the SYMPTOM of the lifestyle. Eat too much processed food and sugar, take a drug to lower your blood sugar, when your body can no longer do the job. The problem isn't the high blood sugar, the problem is the lifestyle that created the high blood sugar. Looking to root cause of problems is one of the primary tenets of Functional Medicine.

A quick story to clarify how medications aren't the answers to lifestyle issues. Let's say you are diagnosed with pre-diabetes and your doctor writes a script for Metformin. He doesn't mention any nutrition changes. The side effects of blood sugar lowering medications, like Metformin, are high blood pressure and diarrhea or irritable bowel syndrome.

So, now you end up going to a gastroenterologist to have a colonoscopy and endoscopy to make sure nothing is really wrong - like a tumor. The Gastroenterologist knows the side effects, but is bound by standards of care to perform the scopes. So, instead of sending you back to your PCP to change meds, or suggesting a lifestyle change, you are told you have Irritable Bowel. Irritable Bowel Syndrome over time creates toxicity and malabsorption issues. Your body is less efficient at absorbing nutrients and becomes toxic from the constipation. Constipation causes stool to back up into the small intestine. Stool doesn't belong here. There are bacteria in the large intestine that do not belong in the small intestine. You get an overgrowth of bacteria in the small intestine, called SIBO, small intestine bacterial overgrowth. This is now treated as an infection. Instead of correcting the blood sugar medication and the constipation. Your doctor puts you on a strong antibiotic. The antibiotic further changes the good bacteria in your large intestine. SIBO has up to a 100% recurrence rate when the antibiotic is taken correctly. (Not the solution) Now you are left with severe bloating, cramping, alternating constipation and diarrhea. AND fatigue from increasing deficiencies, along with the pre-diabetes.

Anyway, up to 60% of diabetics lose an extremity, toes feet, fingers, which increases the need for more antibiotics. Up to 80% end up on dialysis, what kind of life is spending 3 days a week at the dialysis center?

Isn't shifting away from the processed sugar, and unhealthy over-processed foods easier than going through all of this? Isn't eating less processed, whole foods an easier choice? Even if only 90% of the time?

I can't make that make sense, can you? Your body may become malnourished because the diarrhea isn't allowing proper nutrient or water absorption. The diarrhea and constipation that started with the anti-diabetic drugs has now caused high blood pressure because of dehydration from the diarrhea. This is crazy making! You have other options!

High blood pressure medications cause diabetes, or high blood sugar. The circle continues. I will repeat, I am not opposed to remaining on medications while lifestyles are changed. I work with patient's doctors to get them off medications, in an appropriate way. These medications may prolong life, but at what cost to quality of life? What other problems come with these medications? Diabetes is more complicated than just lowering blood sugar. This doesn't mean you have to be a skinny-minny, it doesn't mean you can never eat your favorite snacks or desserts. What about introducing moderation?

To wrap up this little tirade. Pharma is no longer treating one bug with one drug. It's no longer as easy as pill for an ill. Pharma is attempting to treat a complicated biochemical chain of events with a drug that only targets one thing. When the drug breaks into the chain, the rest of the chain continues to run but in a compromised state.

Think about cutting the wire to your Check Engine light. The warning light, the symptom, is gone, but isn't the engine problem still there?

Treating high blood pressure, blood sugar and cholesterol is the same thing. Those symptoms are gone, but the body still has the problem, and inflammation continues, but in a different body part. It shifts the problem somewhere else. All the while, changing to a whole food diet, without processed foods, would solve the problem in the first place. This is considered heretical and alternative to suggest a diet of real foods?!? (mini-rant) OI want to repeat his doesn't mean you have to be a skinny-minny, it doesn't mean you can never eat your favorite snacks or desserts. What about introducing moderation?

Has Pharma made a positive difference? Yes. Of course. But, should it be the first thing we go to when we are suffering from a disease created out of our own lifestyle choices? The fast-easy answer of "take this pill" isn't really a solution, but it has become a societal expectation in America.

Hearing all the commercials on television only heightens this expectation. The more we are told that a pill is the only answer, the more power we give Pharma to run our health. Pharma has no interest in your health, really. The goal of Pharma is to sell drugs and make profits. There is nothing wrong with that either, it's part of the American way. However, as a society, we have been led to believe the drug is the ONLY way to health.

I had a disenchanted patient tell me that "lifestyle" isn't medicine. No, it isn't a drug, that is true. It can actually be more powerful than a drug. It can prevent the need for drugs. I have seen thousands become less dependent and completely free of their prescription medication by controlling their lifestyles. I have seen diabetes, high blood pressure, and high cholesterol plummet with diet and exercise. I have seen auto-immune diseases like rheumatoid arthritis, lupus and

Hashimoto's go into remission with a permanent shift in lifestyle. Prescriptions are NOT a mandatory part of life or aging. You can take that control back and take care of your own health.

Frankly, we are about the only country that doesn't use lifestyle changes as part of the solution to health problems. There are countries with centuries old traditions for healing. Acupuncture, Traditional Chinese Medicine, Ayurvedic Medicine (India), Traditional Herbal Medicine (Germany), Homeopathy (Germany) just to name a few.

You also need to know that Pharma starts indoctrinating doctors as first year medical students. Pharma and education have been long term partners. The academicians are the researchers for these drugs. There is a collaboration between Pharma and large hospitals for clinical trials. The two industries are tightly tied together. The medical schools do not teach nutrition or lifestyle medicine as a general rule. I know, it is appalling. Yes, you will usually know more about nutrition than your medical doctor. According to my research, if medical schools offer nutrition it is a 2-hour elective to a one-month rotation. Most do not have faculty dedicated to training doctors in nutrition. They rely on outside sources and are not invested in teaching even basic nutrition. You have probably spent more than two hours researching this book! This is part of what drove me to go to chiropractic school. Most of the chiropractic programs offer more than 2 years of biochemistry and nutrition, along with laboratory medicine.

Part of my impetus for writing this book is my desire to change the face of healthcare in America. We are really a sick care society. We go to the doctor when we are sick. Doctors are not trained in HEALTH, they are trained in DISEASE recognition.

Honestly, when did changing a diet to less processed foods make anyone sick?

Are there any negative side effects to eating real foods?

Nutrition is necessary for doctors to know. The easy solution is they need to know how to implement programs with their patients. At the very least, they should collaborate with a functional medicine doctor/specialist or health coach who knows how to implement lifestyle changes for patients. As a chiropractic student I had to learn about pharmaceuticals, but the traditional docs don't have to learn about nutrition, does that seem right to you? I am considered the undereducated quack? Hmmm...

Protection

Before I go on, I need to make a disclaimer, I know insurance, and even the most recent iteration the Affordable Healthcare Act, has kept many people from going bankrupt due to medical expenses and has covered surgeries, manifestations of chronic disease, strokes, brain injuries, cancer and many untold tragedies when the patient absolutely would have died without it. I get it! If you want to stop reading my opinion about insurance companies here, please, be my guest. Just skip to the next chapter.

I'll say it again, who pays for care is irrelevant when the basic foundation of the medical education and philosophy is antiquated and broken. It is based in covering for diseases NOT HEALTH.

Would you expect your auto insurance to pay for oil changes or new tires for your car, except if there was a collision?
Would you expect your home owner's insurance to pay for new windows or a new kitchen, except if there was a disaster?

So, please do not expect your insurance to pay for your "HEALTH". It is designed to cover you when disaster strikes. Jim Rohn used to say, "You only have one place to live, you better take care of it." At what point do you have to take personal responsibility for your own body?

What I am about to say is from a doctor's point of view. It is from a point of view where 90% of chronic disease is preventable through lifestyle. My point of view is one where an insurance company doesn't need to interfere or make decisions about what is best for my body. In fact, insurance companies should not be making health care decisions at all. That should be between the doctor and the patient. Yes, I'm trying to keep my rant to a minimum here. They should not be responsible for keeping you healthy either! That is YOUR responsibility. Your homeowner's insurance doesn't pay for a roof or new windows, just as your health insurance isn't going to pay for you to get a plan from your functional medicine doctor, at least not at this time.

Insurance began in the late 1800's and early 1900's to cover miners and railroad workers who got sick or injured to insure Doctors and hospitals would be available. The beginnings of the Blue Cross system gave teachers access to 3 weeks of hospital stay for $6 per year. Insurance was never designed to cover all of our health expenses. It was designed to be there when we are sick. I'm not here to offer a history lesson of the insurance industry, yawn. We got spoiled. Through the years insurance has paid for more and more. I remember time, my mom's vitamins were actually reimbursed by the plan through the plan my dad had through his work. That was the 1970's and 1980's. Then came the invention of the HMO and the PPO and everything changed. By 1992, when I graduated from chiropractic school, everyone had a PPO, the old indemnity plans were gone. Everything was now under the watchful eye of the insurance companies that were starting to lose money through the old indemnity plans. A new era of reporting more information and more control by the insurance companies was in force.

There were a host of reasons for these changes. These tighter controls were in response to hospitals charging outrageous fees for procedures because the insurance company would pay. Pharma got in the mix and expected higher and higher reimbursements for their new, expensive drugs. The US was in an economic downturn and healthcare was a big chunk of our GNP, it was expensive! In order to keep the stockholders happy, reducing healthcare "costs" by tightening amount and who was paid for what procedures was the insurance industries response. At this time, reimbursement for chiropractic care and physical therapy has gone through so many iterations I can't keep track. What I know is, the reimbursement rates are about the same now, as they were in 1992 and some procedures are actually reimbursed less than 1992. Many physical therapists and chiropractors cannot make it in solo practice. Groups are the only way. This forces a change at the Doctor:Patient interface level. You don't always get to see the same doctor, so the relationship is missing. The doctor only has 3-5 minutes to spend with you or he cannot bill enough to justify his existence.

Along with lower reimbursement, more diagnostic testing, and documentation must be done.

Let's talk about diagnostic testing. Testing is paid for all day long by the insurance companies. They even call some of the testing "preventive" like mammograms, colonoscopies and bone density tests.

I believe that these tests have saved lives. I also believe these tests are done unnecessarily much of the time. The Canadian healthcare system won't pay for colonoscopies because they lack proof of saving lives.

Medical malpractice fear forces doctors to run tests to cover their butts, frankly. Your GP, general practitioner, or PCP, primary care physician, is required to send you to a specialist. No longer can your PCP actually manage your care. If they miss something they fear a law suit. It is not good enough for the highly educated doctor to say, "this patient needs treatment because of this issue". Now, a nurse or another doctor at the insurance company, who has never seen the patient, has the power to question the decision, and make a determination about payment. Doctors must spend more time and money to prove what is going on with the patient from an objective stance.

At the same time, reimbursement rates are going down. On day to day issues, minor to moderate injuries, illnesses, and chronic disease like diabetes, heart disease, autoimmune disorders, etc. patients are often ignored or dismissed until something really big shows up on a lab test or X-Ray. Then, the doctor will treat them, because the doctor has to be able to "prove it" to the insurance company that the patient is truly "in need". It has to be "Medically Necessary".

Here's the most appalling part, the person that determines what is medically necessary for the patient is no longer the treating physician. It is someone employed by the insurance company. They have never seen the patient. Yet, they determine whether the treatment is actually necessary. Yes, it's the old saying of putting the fox in charge of the hen house.

I call it "The Insurance Squeeze". The doctor is in the middle, with the patient on the losing end. If the doctor cannot adequately show the insurance company that the patient is sick or needs a particular treatment, reimbursement is not available, and the patient pays out of their pocket or doesn't get care.

From the patient perspective, premiums are at an all-time high, as are copays and out of pocket expenses. They have an expectation that insurance companies have their best interest in mind. This couldn't be further from the truth. Insurance companies hold on to as much money as possible, so they can pay their shareholders and executives. The doctors do all the work and the patient, well, the patient gets nothing except higher premiums, lots of tests, and no real answers as to why their body is sick and no strategies for fixing it.

This is very evident in my practice. I see many patients with Irritable Bowel Syndrome, a disorder where diarrhea can be so urgent, people have to plan their whole day around being close to a bathroom; and constipation can be so severe sometimes a week will go by without a bowel movement. Most of my patients have been told they will just have to live with it!! What? That is crazy. Even gastroenterologists do not recognize the role of diet in gastrointestinal problems. More than once, patients have said their doctor told them it couldn't be food related! How can a gastrointestinal problem NOT be at least partially, food related? Even more infuriating is that if the Gastroenterologist might actually know that food is causing part of the problem, and wants to discuss it with you, he is risking an insurance audit. YES! Offering Lifestyle Counseling is NOT medically necessary! IT IS CRAZY!

There are hundreds of studies linking fast food and sugar and excessive carbohydrate consumption of Americans to the rise in chronic diseases like irritable bowel, diabetes and heart disease. Yet, Doctors risk losing everything if they tell you NOT to eat this or that. Since when did prescribing a sensible diet become NOT medically necessary? There aren't any side effects and it cuts out Pharma. The insurance companies are monitoring his notes, if they see lifestyle counseling, it is deemed "Not Medically Necessary".

I was recently told this story by a local MD. One of the large insurance companies audited his files. Yes, they can request files to make sure we are doing what we are supposed to do. The particular file they chose, the patient was being treated for high cholesterol. The standard of care for high cholesterol is a statin drug which lowers cholesterol. This patient went to this

MD because of symptoms associated with the statin. The MD took the patient off the statin, changed their lifestyle - diet, exercise and stress management. The patient's cholesterol went down as with the medication. However, the Medical Director at the large insurance company said that all the care associated with the lifestyle changes was not medically necessary! The medical director said the patient should have just stayed on the drug. SO, the insurance companies won't pay for lifestyle changes and the drug companies are educating most of our doctors.

Since when is it NOT medically necessary to educate patients about a healthy diet?

This is not the right forum for discussing insurance audits. It is also not the right forum to discuss how the mess was made or who is responsible. But, suffice it to say, the insurance companies, the American Medical Association and Big Pharma have deep pockets, and make the rules. When they don't like the rules, they change the rules. Think IRS audit, but worse. Doctors and patients lose. The insurance company and Pharma are the winners and profit makers.

Patients are left to fend for themselves. They go to Dr. Google and start doing research. They spend hours, days, months and even years educating themselves to the alternatives. When they arrive at their doctor's office, they are told that the research they provided to their doctor isn't relevant, doesn't work, isn't real science and the patient is dismissed and demeaned. Yet, the doctor has less education than the patient at that moment. Doctors won't admit what they don't know, don't have time to do the research because of time constraints of big practices and pressure to see a patient every 3-5 minutes. In order to cover themselves against malpractice, they disregard the patient and hand them a script. The patient feels defeated and angry. They don't know where to turn. The patient is left out of the equation. This is not what medical care is about.

The solution isn't easy. Medical schools don't teach the alternatives, insurance companies won't pay for it, because it "lacks evidence" even though the literature, common sense and antidotal evidence is overwhelming. The American Medical Association has long been after any and all "alternative" practitioners like Naturopaths and Chiropractors. The insurance companies are not unlike the medical schools, they are 50 years behind in their policies and philosophy. So, the patient loses all the way around. Most doctors only have two tools, a Script and a Scalpel.

Go to DrKrisSargent.com for Bonus information about Finding a Functional Medicine Doctor and 6 Key Questions to Ask Your Doctor or Specialist.

Chapter 2: You Need a Team

Health isn't an Accident

Whether you are Madonna, Derek Jeter, or the most amazing person to ever hit the planet (UM...YES, that's you), you need a team. Your support staff may not include media handlers and public relations peeps, but there are some basic components we all need to stay healthy. Think about it. Even your car needs a team. You have to pump the gas and probably refill the washer fluid, maybe even change the oil and air filters. This is general maintenance. But, if you have a collision, you will need specialists for your car. Liken this to what we Eat, Drink, how we Move, Sleep, Think and Feel. These six elements are the body's general maintenance. A heart attack, stroke, cancer or other serious illness is like a collision. You can take care of the basic maintenance on your body, just like you can on your car. It doesn't require a specialist.

Now, if you need something else replaced in your engine, like a belt, transmission fluid, radiator fluid, or spark plugs, you may need the help of a friend who has worked on cars for a long time or maybe a general mechanic. This is still maintenance stuff though. Nothing has gone wrong, it's just a little more complicated.

So, let's say you gain a few pounds over the holidays, even for several years in a row, or have some baby weight and your baby is 12 years old; you want to lose weight and get back in shape. Your Primary Care Physician is not trained in lifestyle medicine. Yes, they will agree you need to lose weight, but most likely won't know what plan or even how to figure out what plan you need.

You can follow some random plan on the internet or you can find a Functional Medicine practitioner. Someone in Functional Medicine will guide you into a sensible eating plan and determine if you need a more specialized diet, like FODMAPS, Grain or Gluten Free, or healthy vegan or vegetarian. I have had a nutrition coach in my office for 10 years! These Physician, practitioners and coaches create a personalized plan for you. This is NOT one-size fits all nutrition. They will take you through understanding how food effects your health, what and how much to eat, when to eat, how much exercise, type and when to exercise, tips on better sleep hygiene, and get your thought process into the optimist and positive psychology you need to be healthy. This is deep maintenance for your body.

Back to our car analogy. What happens if the air conditioner or heater quits working, or you need your brakes replaced? Your car will still run and get you from place to place, but it won't be comfortable, and you might not be able to stop as quickly as you used to, so you will have to be careful. You will probably need a specialist or if you're a gear head you can still take care of these issues on your own. But, these car issues can take some time to fix. This could be similar to pre-diabetes, high cholesterol, irritable bowel syndrome/leaky gut, high blood pressure, hypothyroidism, PMS or heavy periods. Your MD can diagnose any one of these disorders, and even give you some medication. This doesn't really address the root cause of the issue. This is like cutting the wire to the "check engine" light on your dashboard. These are not really diseases. These shifts, high blood sugar, cholesterol and high blood pressure, are shifts in your body chemistry. Your body is trying to compensate for the stress being added to the system and are most likely a response to lack of maintenance. One of the Basic 6 are out of whack. Eat, Drink, Move, Sleep, Think and Feel

- What have you been eating lately?

- Have you consumed 1/2 your weight in ounces of water every day?

- Are you getting exercise 60 minutes 3-4 times per week? Sitting is the new smoking, you will need to move your body even more. I will cover this later.

- Are you sleeping 6-8 hours per night. Women have to get at least 6 hours just to have normal hormone control, more later.

- How is your mental and emotional stress level?

You can solve these conditions, most likely, without medication, or maybe meds for a short time, by fixing your lifestyle. Many "conditions" are really just symptoms that are trying to tell you something is wrong inside your body. You will need someone with some nutritional knowhow to get your lifestyle back on track, and it probably will take some time. Hint: two things proven to create long lasting change in food habits - accountability and logging your food - both easy things to do.

High cholesterol, high blood pressure and high blood sugar are not diseases as we have been led to believe. These are signs that your body trying to cope with some kind of stress. These are symptoms. We can all "live with" these things but life isn't comfortable. If you have seen your primary care physician, they have, most likely, put you on one or more medications that you need to take daily and there are side effects you also have to handle.

Please hear me, there are times when this is necessary!

I have said this several times throughout this book and reiterate here... I totally understand and would never suggest medications should be avoided at all costs. What I am saying is, when you get the first notification that your brakes are going to need to be replaced, does it make sense to make that appointment for that service within the next couple months, so you can plan for that expense and down time for your car? Does it also make sense when we have a symptom or notice something happening in your body, we make a plan to take care of it before something bigger happens? Yes, you may need to use a blood pressure lowering drug for a while, but you do not need to depend on it. You can fix the problem, just like your mechanic can recharge your air conditioner or replace your brake pads without replacing the whole part. You can take control of this lifestyle thing.

Neglecting the squeaky brakes is the same as neglecting symptoms. Taking a medication for the symptom is like putting in ear plugs so you don't hear the squeaky brakes.

What happens when your car collides with something? This is a crisis, an acute issue! It happens suddenly, out of the blue and you generally do not have control over it. You are going to need an expert body guy and mechanic to put your car back together.

In our health analogy, this could be a slip and fall, or other injury, it could be stroke, or heart attack. It could be a serious illness like cancer (although I believe in the team approach for this, more later), strep throat, pneumonia, appendicitis, a urinary tract infection or something acute happens to your body, this is when the medical profession shines! AND, you need a team. Surgery, short term antibiotics, pain medications, and the like are necessary for these, and other, acute situations. When the crisis is over, a healthy lifestyle and your functional medicine team can help you heal. In the realm of cancer, there are specialist emerging in the alternative world who can work with your oncologist, see Cancer Treatment Centers of America.

Hopefully, you can see how keeping your body healthy is like keeping your car healthy.

Symptom or Disease

I am going to take a little side trip and talk about symptoms. Symptoms are the body's way of communicating something is wrong. When we get a headache or stomachache we are supposed to pay attention. We are supposed to notice and not blow it off. When our back or neck and shoulders ache, it is a sign that something inside our body is starting to go awry. Pain is a signal that something is wrong. When we have diarrhea or vomiting, it is a symptom that the body is trying to rid itself of something disagreeable. A fever is there to tell you the body is fighting an infection. Bacteria and viruses live at normal body temperature and perish quicker with a fever.

Our body creates defective cells all the time, these are cancer cells. You are exposed to bacteria, viruses and fungi (like yeast i.e. Candida) every day. Most of the time you don't even know you have been exposed. But, when the body needs to fight something a little stronger or you got a big dose of the bad bugs or toxins, you are alerted by symptoms. Headache, fever, runny nose, sore throat, congestion, muscle aches, bone pain. These are ways your body is telling you something is wrong.

The intelligence of the body is so amazing that when a foreign invader, a bacteria, virus or cancer cell that doesn't belong, the body responds in several ways to kill it. First, your clever body not only recognizes the invader, but starts to produce noxious chemicals to kill invaders, to mark the invaders as the enemy and to summons certain cells to come and fight the invader. The immune system is very complex and wonderful. There is any army inside each of us fighting invaders all the time.

1. The body recognizes bacteria, viruses, fungi and cancer cells because these bad dudes have proteins on their surface that tell the immune system they are invaders. Like a special name tag they are wearing declaring their evil presence. These proteins are known as antigens. All cells have antigens and our body is so cool, it generally knows the difference between what belongs and what doesn't belong. Pretty cool - YEP! I'm geeking out over here. The antigens of the invaders are miraculously recognized by a couple different cells in our body. Macrophages recognize and eat the

invaders. B-Cells make antibodies which are placed on the invader like a flag, so it is tagged for destruction, so the macrophages can see them even better.

2. The body also makes chemicals to help kill off the invaders and cells that don't belong. These chemicals are cellular messages, like email from cell to cell. These messages are called cytokines. Cytokines are part of the communication system of the body, specifically the immune system. Cytokines also create the fever, and the aches you feel. If enough cytokines are made along with other inflammatory substances, you start to feel terrible. They are meant to be temporary, and make you rest. If you sleep and rest, eat good food, stay away from stress your body will repair itself. The invader will be killed, and the cytokines and other inflammatory substances will stop being made. However, if you ignore your symptoms, continue to treat your body as if it had unlimited healing ability even with crappy food, no water, too much caffeine too much stress, you will continue to make these chemicals and you will continue to feel terrible, long after the virus, bacteria fungi or cancer cell has been eliminated. OR, your healing process will be prolonged, leaving you vulnerable to another attack.

3. Stress takes on many forms in our lives. There are some things you may not recognize as stress, but

your body sees it that way. For example, crappy food, lack of water, too much alcohol and or caffeine, lack of exercise, lack of sleep, mental and emotional stress, toxic people, negative outlook. Got the picture? How many stressors do you have in your life? All will break the body down and perpetuate the problem. Your symptoms continue. It is at this point your immune system can get confused. It may start making antibodies to your own cells. This is called an Auto-Immune disorder. In the medical world "auto" means "self". Your immune system is now attacking your own cells. These disorders have names like Hashimoto's disease, Rheumatoid arthritis, lupus, MS and many others. These disorders lead to potentially permanent destruction of tissue. YES! You can turn it OFF, I will tell you how in the upcoming chapters - no worries! And guess what? You probably don't even know this is happening in the beginning. Auto-Immune diseases can start more than 10 years before they are diagnosed. That is why it is so important not to neglect, but respect your body.

When you feel symptoms, the question isn't "where is the ibuprofen?" Well maybe it is, and we will talk about that later, the question is "what is happening in my life to make me feel like this? Have I caught a cold or infection? Did I strain my back moving the couch? Have I been eating good food? Drinking enough water? Getting to the gym? Sleeping enough? What mental and emotional stress is or has been in my life recently, or what is not working in my life? We are going to look at all of these factors and answer all these questions.

Symptoms are not diseases. They are messages from your intelligent body that something is wrong and needs attention. Symptoms are there to warn you. Does it make sense to squash them? Treating the fever, the high blood sugar, the high cholesterol doesn't solve the issue. Besides, each drug has side effects and these side effects are met with other drugs. Treating a fever, prolongs the illness necessitating antibiotics for secondary infections. High blood pressure medication can cause high blood sugar. High cholesterol medications, statins in particular, cause muscle and joint pain, necessitating anti-inflammatories, if your liver can handle it. This is crazy, especially when some simple dietary changes can make a big difference. Just a quick tip right now, cut the starchy carbs and increase vegetables, and watch your cholesterol drop like a rock. I did NOT say anything about red meat. That is not why cholesterol is high. More on this later.

High blood pressure, blood sugar and cholesterol are known to be lifestyle issues, as I have said. Research tells us up to 90% of chronic diseases are lifestyle driven. This is not because of your parents, this is not because you're forced to eat crappy food, or you can't afford vegetables, when you are buying pop and junk for your kids. This is a choice. The popular press even deems the drugs that treat these so-called diseases, Lifestyle Drugs.

Root cause? Lifestyle.

Doesn't it make sense to shift your choices? Does that mean no desserts or sweets, ever again? NO! It means get a handle on your lifestyle once and for all. It means more often than not, making the healthy choice, most of the time, and leaving the sweets alone because you already know they aren't good for you. This isn't a mystery. Seriously, grow up and make positive choices for yourself and your health. You only get one body in this life! It is important! It houses your soul.

Health is the goal, not perfection. Can you carry an extra 10-15 pound and be healthy? Yes, I believe you can, as long as you are creating a healthy lifestyle as you move through your life. Is it better to be at your optimal weight? Of course. Get there on YOUR journey. Long term consistency is more important than attaining the perfect number. Does that mean staying 30+ pound overweight is okay, NO! And no one else is going to tell you, so there it is, the TRUTH!

Health isn't an accident. It's not something that you will eventually "get around to doing". It's a choice, moment by moment, sometimes. Neglecting this one and only vessel that carries your soul, your hopes and dreams, your future health and family is a day by day choice.

Neglect anything long enough and what happens?

You know the answer. Health is something to respect, to take care of like our cars. Most Americans spend more time taking care of their cars than their bodies. There is an easier and different way to do this than waiting for the crisis. Your team needs a good functional medicine practitioner as the pit boss. Check out the resources in the back of the book. You will also need a good chiropractor and physical therapist unless your FM practitioner is one, a dentist, massage therapist, acupuncturist and yes, even traditional MD or DO for the times you need a script or scalpel. When something is wrong, yes, go get all the tests you need, and check in with your Functional doc for nutritional status. Gather your team and let's get it right once and for all! Health is not an accident.

Additional resources are available on DrKrisSargent.com

Chapter 3: But It's So Yummy: CRAP

It's all in Your Head

So far, I have spent a lot of words on explaining the rational reasons to change your lifestyle. My guess is, most of the rational arguments are lost as soon as we start to talk about gooey chocolate cake, candy, your red wine, your entire pot of coffee, the french fries at your favorite restaurant, or the evening binge on potato chips, popcorn (because that's healthy - eye roll), ice-cream, chocolate chips or cookies. This is a general list. What is your go-to emotional stuffing food? How often does this happen to you? I've been there. I get it.

My binge food is and always will be popcorn. I love it. The texture, the crunch, the salt and butter, or parmesan, olive oil and pepper, or pecan oil and Sunny Paris from Penzey's spices, or even crappy movie popcorn with the unidentified yellow liquid called butter flavoring. Mmmmm! YUM! I love it. It reminds me of when I was a kid. My mom always made my sister and I a big bowl of popcorn when her and my dad would leave us with a babysitter. Yep!

Comfort food has an origin. There is a "Root cause" to many of our habits. What is your favorite? How did that particular food become your emotional go to?

I call this type emotional eating the Triple Threat.

First, it has to do with the original emotion that pushed you to the limit. Whether it's the habit of relaxing with food, or binging because you had a bad day, you feel bad, scared, lonely, shameful, angry about something. OR you like to celebrate with food. Most of us celebrate with food and cry with food. In any case when you use food in any way other than to nourish your body you are Emotional Eating. This emotion is the first part of the triple threat. Emotions are made out to be the bad guy here. So, here is the truth about our emotions.

Our emotions are created by energy preceding a chemical release in our body. Therefore, emotions are just energy in motion, that create a feeling. Research tells us that this energy will only last about 90 seconds. If you can just hang on for a minute and a half, your emotions are likely to change. Come on, you can do anything for 90 seconds. So, our emotions become the first of the Triple Threat. The second threat is the crappy food we generally choose to binge on. You know what that is don't you? I will not list the myriad of binge foods my patients have told me about. You already know mine, popcorn.

So, you eat the Binge Food. Now you feel emotional about the original reason and feel bad about the food. Feeling bad or guilty about eating the food is the second Threat. AND most likely, your body feels horrible too. You feel sluggish, full, bloated or any number of physical symptoms common to binging - the third member of the Triple Threat. You end up feeling emotionally crappy about two things and physically crappy from the CRAP you just ate. UUUGGGHHH!

The cycle starts over and over out of habit. You can control it. REALLY! You can. We will discuss even more strategies later. This is NOT JUST about will power either! Most of us have what is known as "decision fatigue" by some point in our day. It's that fatigue that determines your ability to "just say no" to the habits of eating CRAP instead of dealing with the emotions.

There were several times in my life, popcorn took over and became the only emotional outlet. Once when I was young, I made a really bad relationship decision. I moved to Manhattan, yes New York City, without friends or family. Popcorn was my best friend. There were several times during Chiropractic school when the stress of professional school got the best of me. Popcorn was my go-to stress reliever. You get the picture. I am not perfect! Geez! I would have nothing to write about...how boring life would be if we were all perfect!

Even with my strong commitment to health. I have always worked out, and mostly eaten smart. The weight thing and fear of not being liked or accepted because I was fat, has generally driven me to make the healthy choices. Maybe not healthy motivations...but...Fear can create positive shifts...Emotional eating was still an issue. It did seem uncontrollable. I actually didn't understand it. It took years of reading and being fully aware of my behavior before I could make the change. A new habit emerged from my research. Stop, Challenge, Choose - thank you Dr. Wayne Scott Andersen and Mel Robbins.

First, a technique that does not rely on talking myself out of it, a technique that does not deprive me, or allow my emotions to go unvalidated. I learned to count. Yep. Count.

I counted backwards from 10. Ten little seconds. When I would pull out the microwave popcorn or the popcorn maker, I would stop myself at some point in the process. Well, most of the time. Sometimes I didn't catch on until the deed was done and I was shoving popcorn in my face. But, when I would realize what I was doing I counted backwards from 10 - STOP. I would take that 10 seconds and I would acknowledge the emotion or Challenge and the Challenge of the popcorn.

What had happened that was so bad that I was punishing myself by gorging on popcorn? This challenge of your own behavior serves to create more and more awareness. It also takes up that 90 seconds of feeling the energy in motion of your emotions.

I also asked myself if I was in my appropriate weight zone - plus or minus 2 pounds from my weight goal. For me, bouncing between about 142-145 is great. Remember I said, "FOR ME". Each of us has to determine where we feel good and look our best. Using the BMI charts can be helpful.

Back to the process already. I would really tune in to my heart and intuition. I would promise myself that if this issue was still bothering me on the upcoming weekend, I could have the popcorn then; OR if something happened on a weekend, I would pick a random day in the next week. This is a CHOICE. I would delay my tasty, salty crunchfest. I would then put away all the instruments of debauchery, the popcorn maker or little hard bag I was going to put in the microwave and do something else. ANYTHING else!!

Take a walk if it was nice, take a bath, read a book or any number of things I could possibly think of to shift my focus. I use this for any and every bad habit - including anxiety and worry. This is when I learned to journal. Putting the incidents down helped me come to a clearer understanding of why I had jumped at the chance to make myself fat. The very thing I feared the most. YOU CAN TOTALLY DO THIS!!

I made a decision. I made the decision that I would be in control of my emotions. I would no longer be controlled by the fleeting feelings of despair, loneliness, exhaustion, boredom, stress of the day or situations that were not in my control. These feelings were just energy in motion that can dissipate in 90 seconds, if I let them. Food is not the way out of any of those emotions. Sitting in those emotions, feeling through them, writing them down and learning that fear, shame, or vulnerability was attached to the binge.

This created a monumental shift. This habit led me to write this book. I had tried other times. Fear, shame and vulnerability stopped me. But not this time!

Sitting in those emotions one day with my website developer, I came up with the acronym CRAP. Not only does it describe how you feel, physically and emotionally, but also describes most of the Standard American Diet (SAD), Modern Urban Diet (MUD) and the foods we chose to binge on when we feel that way. It's not only how we feel physically mentally and emotionally it's what we end up feeding those feelings, and how we feel afterward. Right? And so, it goes:

> You have a crappy day, so you reward yourself with your favorite binge food. Then you feel even worse! Here's the thing, you actually lose three times, right? The Triple Threat. First, you had

a bad day, something happened to upset you, you let it control you - CRAP - so, #2 you binged which equals "bad for you food" - CRAP - and the physical manifestations - CRAP, #3 You punish yourself mentally and emotionally - CRAP- for binging, and harangue yourself mercilessly until you start the cycle all over again, or vow you will never binge again, until you break that promise and so it goes. This is crazy making! You are only learning to NOT trust yourself. Breaking out of this loop requires some serious work. You CAN DO THIS - you will discover what has kept you stuck in your life - and not just around food! It's awesomely freeing!

CRAP is now going to help you. No longer will this word be a negative! It will be a path out of all the craziness, the illnesses, the weight issues, the irritable bowel, hormone mess and PMS. You will go from Crapulous to Fabulous!

What does CRAP mean?

C stands for <u>Clean It Up</u>. Clean up your lifestyle. What are you Eating? Drinking? How are you Moving,

Sleeping, Thinking and Feeling? These represent the foundation of your health. Supplements cannot cover up a CRAPPY lifestyle. Medication is also not a magic pill as I have shown you. This does not mean broccoli and chicken for the rest of your life either. Frankly, my family will barely eat chicken. We are carnivores and eat a lot of red meat, as clean as I can find and afford. We eat pork, bison, and lamb. I am not opposed to being a vegan, and I eat a lot of raw veggies and a few nuts. Yes, I eat popcorn and key lime pie as a treat, when my weight is in a 2-pound zone of where I want it to be. That is part of my decision-making tree, for treating myself. When I say CLEAN - I mean 90-95% of the time. That may leave a little wiggle room for one indiscretion a week when you are staring out. Depending on what your body needs and how long it takes to heal, those indiscretions may be a little more often if you can maintain your health. I will go through a comprehensive program to tackle each of these areas of your life.

R stands for get to the <u>Root and Restore Function</u>. There are seven basic functions of the body: Communication, Structural, Assimilation, Defense and Repair, Energy production, Biotransformation and Elimination, and Transportation. When those functions are disrupted by our poor lifestyles, symptoms manifest. In order to fix the root cause, the DYS-Function must be addressed at the core. This is called getting into Root Cause healing solutions. You will need some intensive nutrition for six months to two years, depending on the chronicity of your issues. I know it seems like a long time. Look at the last 6 months, lots has happened and think about how fast it went…

How long have you felt poorly?

When was the last time you recall feeling healthy, vibrant, able to think clearly, and get your to-do list accomplished?

I will outline Basic and Comprehensive Gut Healing Protocols including Heal Your Leaky Gut and Irritable Bowel, Balance the Immune System, Detoxify and Regenerate the Liver Protocols, Awaken Your Adrenals and Harmonize Your Hormones. These will heal you from the inside, out.

A stands for <u>Action, Apply, Ask, and Awareness.</u> Action is the difference between a dream and a goal. You can want something really bad, meditate on it, pray for it, wish for it, see yourself there, but until you take the first step, you are stuck in your day dreams.

Action is about application. Apply what you are about to learn. Constantly Ask yourself where you are in the process. This creates Awareness.

This is the place where self-help books get a bad reputation. This is where "diets don't work" comes from… all the BS in most of these books works if the advice is followed, even at 80-90%!

When you get stuck ask yourself what is missing in your plan? Maybe you went to a birthday party, had some cake and didn't feel too bad so you brought back sugar, slowly, in small quantities that over the past few weeks have grown into larger quantities.

Getting in the habit of asking yourself "<u>what am I doing?</u>", then start tracking your habits again. You will unearth the root of your "sudden" 5-pound weight gain, return of stomach issues, etc. We often underestimate the power of stressful events in our life. There is a strong mind-body connection. It's so strong, our gut is called our second brain. Events in our lives, even happy events like a graduation or a move, influence our health in ways that we don't always understand.

Attitude is also important. What is your typical attitude through your day? Have you noticed the words coming out of your mouth? Complaints or compliments? Attitude IS A CHOICE!

I will be show you a systematic way to ask yourself what is going on, so you can stay in touch with your body, and then apply what you know to get back on track. Act, Apply Ask… rinse and repeat…

P stands for Personalized Plan. Functional Medicine is all about a personalized approach. Discovering what works for you is part of the journey. There will be many tried and true solutions in this book. Some will work for you, some won't. You will be able to personalize your solution.

Take this process personally! This IS ABOUT YOU! What are you doing for YOU? Who is surrounding you? Are they supportive? We become the 5 people we hang around with most of the time. SO, what does your personal life look like?

I also like to think of the P as Patience in the Process; Procrastination and Perfectionism are not welcome. The old adage that life is about the journey is overused and makes me roll my eyes and maybe even throw up a little in my mouth. Even though I understand it, I am a goal-oriented girl. Once I make a decision, I want it DONE. Unfortunately, that is also a place of getting stuck in wanting it to be done, but not actually taking the action to make it happen. So, YES, I understand the frustration of the PROCESS. Yet it remains, staring you, and I, in the face. One foot in front of the other, most of you will want to start with baby steps. Some of you will take the bull by the horns and never look back.

Think about this: look at the previous 6 months. List out at least 10 things that have happened in your life in the last 6 months. Holidays, kids, friends, nieces and nephews, sisters, brothers, family, friends, events, travels, cars, appliances, weather related items - just a few things to get you thinking. Look at the calendar 6 months ago. Can you believe all the stuff that happened? CRAP! I know, RIGHT?

One more note on time. Do you know how many times I hear "I am too busy" to eat, plan meals, take time to eat or drink water. All of that is up to you! Seriously folks, you can choose what you do with each and every second you spend on the planet. Do a time audit. For one week, write down how much time you spend doing everything. I know it's a pain in the ass.

Do you want to be "too busy" until you have that major health crisis - that is fine too? What are you doing with your time? Social Media? Shopping? Working too much overtime? Doing too much for your kids? Spouse? Parents? Watching television or YouTube? When is your health going to disrupt everything you're doing? When are you going to say, "NO!"? When are you going to take back 4-5 hours a week for yourself?

Your next 6 months will be just as full, AND you can be healing your body at the same time.

To use an old Jim Rohn quote: "Why? Why do you want to change your health? Why Not? That is the best answer. Why Not You? How long will you wait? Why Not Now? What are you waiting for? You are literally one healthy snack or meal away from a lifetime of good or bad health - you chose."

CRAP! It is just so fitting... It's how you feel, what you say about how you feel, what the typical American is eating that created part of the problem... and no one likes to talk about it!

The rest of this book is going to outline how to heal your body and go from feeling Crapulous to Fabulous!

Chapter 4: C: Clean it Up
Eat, Drink, Move, Sleep, Think and Feel

This is here most of us get stuck isn't it? First of all, give yourself a break. With so much information out there, it is difficult to discern what is real, what works and what is BS. Second, the key is to figure out what works for YOU! We are all different genetically, physically, spiritually, mentally, and emotionally. Our bodies do not always read the rules about what foods make us feel good or not. What is supposed to be "good for you", may not always be good for YOU! What works for your friend, may not work for you.

Patients tell me all the time how they went on the latest internet diet and felt great! Yeah, I was Paleo for about three months, or I did a Whole 30 and my skin, hair, stomach, joints, etc., felt great. I lost weight, it was amazing. But then I went on vacation and I haven't been able to get back to it. It's so much work, and it's too restrictive. Now, I am starting to feel terrible again, I guess it didn't work and I don't know what to do next.

UM, your body told you exactly what it needed.

Were you paying attention? You felt better eating cleaner! Did you miss it? Or, did you think your body that was sick for the past however many years would be healed enough to go back to the Standard American Diet (SAD MUD) of poison? You cleaned out the poison and felt great, when you went back to the poison you felt horrible again? Resolve to NEVER go back to a regular diet of the CRAP! Yes, you may be able to indulge at times, but can we agree to let your body heal first? And for a while? Yes, like 6 months to a year... Clean up the BAD CRAP and get to the GOOD CRAP in life. Hmmmmm??

So, let's get real for a minute, you actually know exactly what to do! You may not like it, but you know what to do. If a certain plan works for you, it alleviates your symptoms, and you have energy and the best sex of your life? Then, what is the problem? I believe the problem resides in a few places.

1. We feel deprived. We live with a habit of food rewards for everything from depression to celebration. Success in the food arena takes awareness and adding in some new habits. You can continue to be an emotional eater, or not. You can choose some different habits around food. It starts out with a game that becomes a habit. The new habit of delayed gratification. Let's say I have a horrible day at work and come home to find my kids fighting and the dogs chewing on my favorite shoes. UGH! Dinner isn't ready, so it would be easy

to make some popcorn or pizza and call it a night. Right? And then how would that feel tomorrow? Crapulous! So, instead, I count from 10, remind myself I can indulge a little on the weekend, but tonight I am making salads for everyone. When the weekend rolls around, more often than not I have forgotten about the stressful day and the popcorn, or don't want it. And how do I feel about the salad night? FABULOUS! You can create this or similar system so you don't feel deprived.

2. We don't stick to something long enough to allow our body to heal. We get sucked into thinking we should be well in a week or 30 days, then we can go back to eating CRAP again. In Hashimoto's The Root Cause by Izabela Wentz, she says it took her two years to heal, and she is still gluten free for life. Healing takes time. This happened to me too! I was almost 40 years old when I started having children! No issues getting pregnant - for that I am very grateful, however, the post part depression and weight gain that ensued was horrendous. My thyroid, ovaries and adrenals were a mess. I had my daughter at almost 39 years old and my son at almost 41 - it took me until I was 45 to feel right again! Then I still had 40 pounds to lose! Postpartum depression happens in and to all of our cells. It's not just the brain involved in depression or the adrenals in adrenal fatigue syndrome. It's not just the thyroid involved in thyroid disease. It's not just the GI tract involved in abdominal

pain. The whole body suffers. So, the whole body has to heal.

Let me say this again. The WHOLE body has to heal. I see this all the time. A patient has been on supplements for a couple months and nothing has changed. Two things are going on and I have to ask. Are you cleaning up the food or just taking supplements? Are the supplements professional grade or are you taking the cheapest thing you can find? Not all supplements are created equal. Professional brands are like pharmaceuticals. Ingredients are tested for quality and substances. Ingredients are tested for toxins that don't belong in your supplements. The companies that really care about you getting healthy, also care about their supplements containing the most active and highest quality ingredients. Ys, you will pay a little more for them. But, if the supplement you are buying, isn't helping, you are wasting your money. Become a patient or enroll in my online DIY program. Have your Functional health panel blood work done, get your full deficiency report, then you will know whether your supplements are working or not.

We are programmed to believe that the antibiotic cures us of the infection. Pill for an ill and we are all better in a week. Right??? Not really. Yes, it helps, but ultimately, it's the job of our immune system to bring those bad bugs to justice and kill them. It seems to only take a week or 10 days, but the healing goes beyond the 10 days. You have to stick with the healing plan 95-100% in the beginning, knowing that it won't be forever! You will have to remind yourself that lifestyle changes will have to be followed more for the first 6-12 months.

3. We don't see the success we are having through the busyness of our lives. If you have not measured yourself in any way except pounds, you are probably missing some fundamental data. If you are trying to lose weight, are your clothes getting too big even though the scale isn't moving? How is your skin? Hair? Nails? Periods? Moods? How is the quality of your sleep? There is a lot of data we miss because we simply are not in touch with our bodies and our health. Make sure you take my Metabolic Screening Questionnaire found on my website DrKrisSargent.com

4. We really do not believe that what we eat makes a difference to our health. We don't believe lifestyle makes any difference. While we are pulling out old clichés, you are what you eat, seriously think about that statement. What are your new cells made of? Fast food, devoid of nutrients? What kind of cell would that kind of CRAP make? Do you think if you eat CRAP you will get a healthy body? What

kind of neurotransmitters will you make - the chemicals responsible for making you brain and nervous system function? What kind of healing will you get? Okay, so vitamin and mineral deficiencies are real. Vitamin deficiencies create symptoms. Doctors can give you a script for the symptom or you can really find out the underlying Root Cause. Almost every single patient I see is somewhat deficient in iron, B-12 and vitamin D, and most are dehydrated, despite drinking a lot of water. I will address this issue later.

5. You don't realize that when you clean up your diet, you aren't just effecting your gut, thyroid or whatever body part you think is sick, you are effecting your whole body. When you take the CRAP out and put the good stuff in, your whole body will benefit!! Your whole body starts to heal. Your gut first, then immune system, liver, adrenals, hormones, neurotransmitters, ALL of it.

So Doc, what do I eat?

Good question! Let's look at macronutrients and what each one does for the body.

Protein: Proteins are actually made from combining molecules called amino acids. There are 20 different amino acids. Protein can come from animal or plant sources. Chicken, fish, beef, bison, lamb venison, turkey, you get the picture. These are animal proteins. Animal proteins are considered "complete proteins" because they contain all of the essential amino acids necessary for the body. Cheese is a protein and a fat. Milk is a protein, carbohydrate and a fat. Plant sources of protein do not always contain all of the essential amino acids and in a true vegetarian/vegan lifestyle, legumes, or beans, need to be combined with a grain, like corn or rice, to have the full complement of all 20 amino acids. Yes, that carries a significant number of carbohydrates and calories to the vegetarian/vegan lifestyle. I want to be clear. I am not opposed to the vegetarian or vegan lifestyle. That being said, it is very difficult for many of my patients to lose weight, maintain weight, keep their blood sugar even, and have normal cholesterol levels when they are on a vegetarian or vegan diet because of the higher carbohydrate content needs to get all the amino acids necessary for a healthy body.

Carbohydrates: Carbohydrates are made from combining single glucose(sugar) molecules together in long chains. The denser the chain, as in grains and starchy vegetables (root vegetables like potatoes, turnips, beets, even the beloved sweet potato), the more carbohydrates the food will contain. Grains, fruits and vegetables are natural sources of carbohydrates.

Does it make sense to eat real food? I have several plans I use through my association with the Institute of Functional Medicine, I have also created E4E, Eat for Energy, to get you started. The outline is in this chapter.

Energy, blood sugar and food are intimately connected. Keeping your blood sugar even is crucial to Cleaning It Up! Blood sugar imbalances create the following symptoms:
- morning and afternoon crashes 10-11am and 2-4 in the afternoon
- irritability
- anxiety
- lack of focus and concentration
- memory issues
- increased inflammation associated with everything from joint pain to Autoimmune disorders
- Hormone problems like PCOS (women with facial hair, infertility, horrible periods) and low testosterone in men (yes man boobs and erectile dysfunction)
- Irritable bowel
- Candida and yeast infections
- Weight/fat gain
- High Cortisol, the stress hormone is released when you skip meals, or freak out about something turning on muscle burning and adding fat.
- and more...

Like I said, this is the MOST important step in cleaning up your diet, and your body.
Following this plan of real food for 90 days will be a game changer. These food choices optimize blood sugar and energy levels by keeping your tank full of nutritionally dense foods. Ladies eat the smaller portions, Gentlemen eat the larger portions.

Choose ONE of the options:

Breakfast: (choose one option)
1-2 eggs/ 1 cup berries

1-2 eggs w/ vegetables
Turkey sausage/1 egg/ 1/2 apple
1C Plain Greek Yogurt, stevia and 1 C Berries

Mid-Morning Snack
20 almonds OR 20 cashews OR 10 walnuts with raw vegetables
1/4C Hummus with raw vegetables

Lunch
2-4C salad 2-4 oz protein
Vegetables(2C) and 3-4 oz protein, 1/4 C rice/legumes(beans)
Same as breakfast choices

Mid Afternoon Snack
2 T peanut /almond butter and small apple
1/4 C Guacamole (or 1/4 avocado) with raw vegetables
Same as mid-morning
1 Cheese stick or Babybel with a small apple or 1/2 C berries

Dinner
4-6 oz Protein, 3 C vegetables (no corn), 1/3 C sweet potato OR rice OR legumes

Vegetables - These provide more fiber for keeping you full and keeping bowel movements normalized; they also provide fuel for the good bacteria. You may choose ANY non-starchy vegetable. The starchy vegetables in general are potatoes. You can choose small amounts of other root vegetables in place of the sweet potato.

Fruit - Limited to 2 servings per day. Although fruit is packed with great nutrients, it is also packed with sugar, which at this point serves to feed the bad bacteria and yeast. This is contrary to our goal of creating a healthier intestinal environment. The sugar also serves to increase insulin release which can create inflammation.

Protein - preferably lean cuts of chicken, turkey, beef, pork, fish, shellfish, venison, or buffalo. Any protein you like will suffice. Do not fry it. Protein serves to slow the release of blood sugar into the blood stream, as well as provide the amino acids necessary for detoxification enzymes and muscle maintenance.

Blood Sugar

Blood sugar maintenance can make or break an entire program. Eating Paleo or AIP is awesome, but if you are not eating every 4 hours or so, your blood sugar will drop. Low or high blood sugar will result in symptoms I mentioned earlier. Yes, there are some great fasting programs by Dr. Jason Fung, I will not address those here.

The dark line shows what happens when we decide donuts and oatmeal are a good idea for breakfast. If you eat at 8 in the morning you crash around 10-10:30, about 2-2.5 hours later. And you grab for the glucose, or a coffee with sugar and a granola bar. The same thing happens in the afternoon when you eat a high carb low nutrient lunch. You get sleepy and unproductive between 2 and 4 in the afternoon. So, you grab for the glucose again, maybe another coffee or some kind of sugary snack and the roller coaster starts again. At the top of the line, glucose starts doing damage to small blood vessels, resulting in blindness, diabetic neuropathy, loss of circulation in your hands and feet with a decreased ability to heal and kidney damage, just to mention a few of the most common diabetic issues that happen over time.

ALSO, the hormonal impact for females is that your estrogen will shift to testosterone production causing period disruption, or PCOS, polycystic ovarian syndrome, mood swings, hair growth where you don't want it (ewww!) and PMS at the very least. For men, testosterone shifts to estrogen production, weight gain, man boobs and small balls result, not super attractive, guys. At the same time, insulin is trying to bring the glucose back down by shuttling it into your cells. When we eat highly processed high carbohydrate foods (chips, cookies, donuts, deserts, pasta, bread, granola bars, yogurt), your body requires more and more insulin. So much, that your body stops recognizing it efficiently. This is insulin resistance.

Crash and Crave
Glucose Grab

Unless you are training for a marathon, your body cannot possible use this much sugar. Yes, those "carbs" turn into sugar, glucose, for the body to use as fuel. However, because we don't usually exert that much activity, there is an excess of glucose. Simply put, insulin will shove as much in the cells as possible, then the liver will take over and turn the excess sugar into triglycerides and fat. That fat gets stored in your least favorite places! You know where those places are... your belly or butt! BUT, the bigger issue is when fat is stored between your organs. This is known as VAT, visceral adipose tissue. VAT

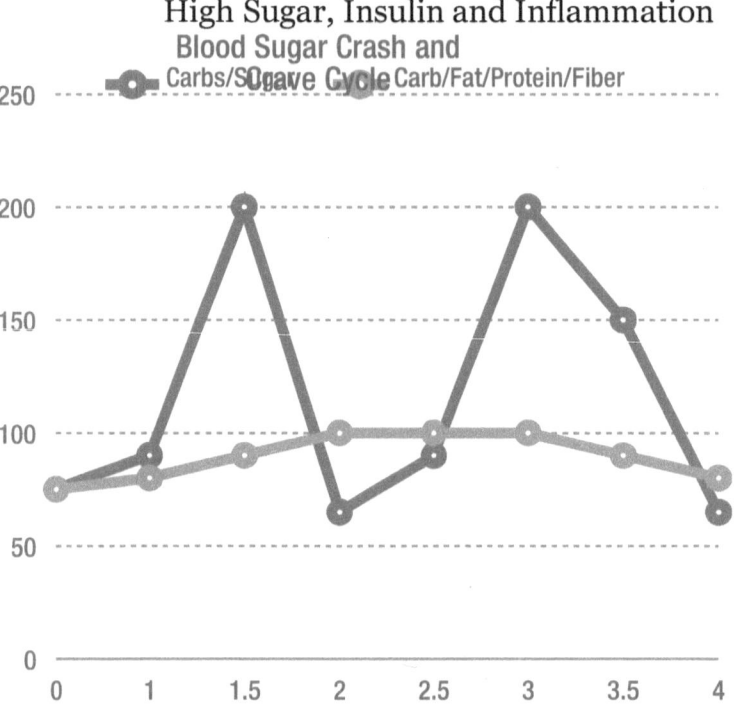

creates even more inflammation and hormone disruption starts. Your liver can also get fat, called fatty liver disease or non-alcoholic fatty liver (NAFL).

So, what? You get fat... AND all of this fooling around with glucose levels creates inflammation which can lead to autoimmune diseases, joint pain, foggy brain, achy muscles, fibromyalgia, adrenal fatigue, and of course, diabetes. You name it, when you do not control your blood sugar, it will take over and make you sick. All of that happens at the top of the darker line of the curve.

When your blood sugar finally crashes, you start craving. At the bottom of the curve, your body makes cortisol to bring your blood sugar back up and you generally eat something, so you overdo it again, causing another rise in the glucose and the cycle starts all over.

When you skip meals, cortisol will also come to the rescue, breaking down muscle tissue, a huge chunk of your metabolism, to raise your blood sugar. YES, skipping meals causes muscle break down or wasting called sarcopenia. This is the last thing you want to happen to your body. Muscle wasting, or sarcopenia is a leading indicator of mortality. Sarcopenia is not compatible with longevity. This is where the cravings you seemingly cannot control are started. So, you reach for the next carb and you are rolling again. All day long your blood sugar rises and falls. It wreaks havoc on your energy, mood and hormones.

Cortisol is viewed as a stress hormone by your body. It is made in your adrenal glands. When your body is under this kind of stress over time, it causes adrenal fatigue. Basically, these life stressors, whether food, alcohol, negative people, relationships, etc., are viewed by the body as a tiger chasing us through the wild. Our body is designed well to handle short term stressors for survival. Blood flow changes from digestion and rest to our big muscles, lungs and heart so we can run away. When life was slower and simpler, or if you are a zebra on the plains in Africa, the stress of a tiger chasing you ends shortly. You are either dead, or you get away, then you get to shake off the stress and chill. However, in our crazy American lifestyle, we never stop. Every day we get up and start running from that tiger. Whether it's bills or the boss, kids, friends, significant others or putting crappy food in our face, we are under siege. Do you think your body can digest foods (hello GERD), make normal enzymes and hormones, have a sex drive and get pregnant when it thinks it's being chased all day by a tiger? Really, you think your body cares about any of this when it is being chased by a tiger?

Please understand, today's stress lifestyle is the main cause of disease, lost wages, higher insurance premiums and premature aging in this country. These are all habits of the choices we make. Radical as it may seem, especially given the societal pressure to be rich and famous, to do more and more, have more and more etc., there are ways out of your situation. We will get into this later. For now, just know there are options you may not have considered. Yes, you can down size, change jobs, find a different path. Start with changing what you have control over. You can control what you eat and drink, how you move sleep, think and feel.

When your body is stressed, creating cortisol, digestive enzymes and stomach acid are not produced properly. Bloating, feeling full, reflux or heartburn known as GERD, gassy, irritable bowel can result. This turns into Leaky Gut, then the Immune system is negatively influenced, inflammation begins. Other issues will manifest.

On the graph, the lighter line represents a balanced meal of fat carbs and protein with a little fiber. When you add protein, a small amount of water and fiber to the carbs, like an egg plus 1/3 C cooked oatmeal, you have a completely different outcome. See the E4E plan above. That is a simple place to start. Smaller portion of sugar plus protein and fat/fiber cause a slower release of glucose into your blood stream. So, your energy lasts longer. You no longer crash and crave, and you have even energy for 3.5-4 hours. Your body doesn't store fat or have the need to produce cortisol. If you eat small meals like this throughout the day, your energy will stay even, and you will not crash and crave. Your moods and brain fog will improve. Over time, lower inflammation will lead to less symptoms... It will take about three to five days to get this going and under control and will take about 3-6 months really start seeing the full effect of healing. It took me 4 years to heal my immune system and blood sugar issues after I had my kids at 40 years old... You will FEEL better quickly, within a couple weeks or sooner, but healing long standing adrenal, thyroid, blood sugar, and weight issues takes time.

I think the important part of eating clean is understanding the need to portion control your food. Eating Paleo isn't a reason to eat an entire pound of bacon, or a 16-ounce steak. Let's look at label reading. In order to really figure out the portion control you will need to attain and or maintain a proper weight, reading labels is crucial. Let's talk about macro's. I have a YouTube video about reading labels and getting a good balance of carbs and proteins. To keep it simple, keep your carbs and proteins at a 1 to 1 ratio, never more than 2 to 1. In other words, if an item has 10 grams of carbs, it needs to be balanced with 5-10 grams of protein. This alone will be a game changer. If you are female, do not consume more than about 20 grams of carbs at one time. Use an app to help you learn carb amounts. My Fitness Pal is my favorite.

So, what about all those magic shakes that people are selling to help you lose weight? There is a time for meal replacements. Carrying an excessive amount of weight is not healthy in anyone's book. The right meal replacements can take the place of some food, teaching portion control, and getting glucose in order, all the while allowing the person some quicker weight loss than the typical diet. This also allows the person to understand their relationship with food. When food is replaced with shakes, bars, soups etc. all portion controlled. You are forced to deal with any emotional issues you may be using food to numb. I use a very specific program in my office.

Drink

Our body is comprised of over 80% water. We hear we should drink water, but most of us seldom drink enough. The formula is 1/2 of your weight in ounces. If you weigh 100 pounds, drinking 50 ounces is adequate. Why? Maybe you know that you should drink more water but never really understood WHY.

1. When our cells make energy, the molecules of hydrogen and oxygen are necessary for that process. So, dehydration often equals fatigue.

2. Many people crave carbohydrates or sugar, this is often just a misinterpretation of the thirst signal. Next time you are craving, grab a dill pickle, 3 olives or some celery and some water. Wait 30 minutes. I bet the crave goes away.

3. Water hydrates joints and skin. More water, ladies, equals less wrinkles.

4. It allows your body to detoxify itself. Think about a swamp or a bog, no fresh spring here, just like a big mud puddle with all kinds of unfriendly critters. This is what happens inside your body when you don't drink enough water. It becomes stagnant

and smelly. When there is a fresh source of water, the gunk goes away.

5. Our brain floats in something called cerebrospinal fluid. It is mostly water. Really, you want to mess with your brain?

6. Muscle cramping and intestinal cramping. Your muscles are not just around your bones. Your heart is a muscle, and there is smooth muscle in your gut and your uterus, ladies. Menstrual cramps anyone? Stomach or intestinal cramping Without proper hydration, muscles cramp up, causing pain and discomfort. This alone may be a big part of your digestive issue, if you have irritable bowel syndrome.

7. You blood is also over 1/2 water. It allows your body to carry the proteins, vitamins and other nutrients around your body.

I want to talk about coffee and alcohol a little here and then again in the sleep section. Many people use caffeine to wake up in the morning and alcohol to get to sleep. We have become a nation of overweight, exhausted, addicted multitaskers. Caffeinating your way through the day causes dehydration and increased cortisol production. This is the stress hormone that makes you fatter by breaking down your muscle tissue. Caffeine messes with your blood sugar (didn't I just carefully outline why blood sugar maintenance is so important?), which in turn messes with your energy and ability to sleep. Not to mention it is a stimulant which is a drug and has side effects. Like irritability. And you wonder why you are tired and crabby all the time.

Clean it up entails cutting back on the caffeine and alcohol. I didn't say none. But, seriously, a pot of coffee and a bottle of wine a day might signal you have an issue!

Water is boring, yes. But it doesn't have to be boring. You can put any number of fruits - lemon or melon; vegetables - cucumbers and even herbs - mint, thyme, basil, in your water to make it more fun. Check out my website for more fun water ideas, www.DrKrisSargent.com. You can download Fun Water Ideas.

Move

Move has several meanings. First, move your body, second, move your bowels and third, get your spine adjusted.

Sitting is the new smoking. It is bad for us, we know it, it is addictive, and we keep doing it! Stop sitting! Move your body at least 30 minutes per day. Yes, park your car in the far part of the parking lot, walk up the stairs instead of the escalator or elevator, go to the water cooler or restroom on a different floor of your office building, do exercises at your desk. ANYTHING! There are apps for your phone, iPhone and Android, and for your computer, Mac and PC that will remind you to take a break and even offer suggestions for exercises. Many of these apps are free, so, no excuse not to try one.

We have muscles to move our joints and hold us up. We have core muscles that stabilize our entire body as we move. We need to keep them strong if we are to live a long and healthy life. Moving our body prevents strokes, heart attacks and falls on the ice. You can start by walking out to your mailbox, or down the hallway to the next apartment. You don't need fancy shoes to get started. However, you will need new shoes every 6 months or so, even if they are relatively expensive. Your feet and joints will thank you for the extra cushion. Unfortunately, the insides of our shoes wear out long before the outsides lose their luster. Walk anywhere you can be safe. There are malls that open early for walkers, there are plenty of great country roads, get a bright yellow or orange vest so you will be visible, and city neighborhoods make great places to walk even if you have to take a bus to a safer area. Move your body!

Yes, you can get a personal trainer. That is optimal, but not necessary. The local YMCA, Park District, gym or Jazzercise class will be fine.

You can find everything you need on YouTube actually. Some cable companies have exercise shows On-Demand, or you can record them. But, if you have a smart phone, YouTube has plenty to get you started without any special equipment.

I have taken out every excuse except, "I do not have time". Now, you are going to hear the truth, and you may not like it. You may be mad and close this book. However, I can tell what a person values can be found on their bank statement and their calendar. If it is more important to go shopping for something useless, spend time on social media, volunteer for every school project for your kids, say yes to every request at church, you get the picture, then you are correct, you do not have time. However, if health is a part of what you want to teach your family, or is important to you, you can find the time.

Solution: Chart every activity every minute of every day for a week. Yes, including your shower and personal time. It's like charting your food. When you realize what you are doing with your time, you will realize there are some changes you can make. You will find time wasted on figuring out what someone will think about you if you wear such and such, or if your hair isn't just right, social media, shopping for stuff you don't "need", this is time that can be rearranged.

We all have 24 hours a day. We all only come around in this life once. What are you going to do with the time given? In the bigger, existential conversation, how do you want to spend your life on earth? Living a long healthy productive life with a healthy body like a race car or basically becoming a jalopy on the side of the road?

Move your bowels. If you are not pooping every day, we need to change that as soon as possible! Normal for you may be once a week and that is common, but it is far from healthy. Think about leaving your trash in the kitchen for a week. Or, think about not turning on the garbage disposal in the sink after dinner for a week. Disgusting, right?! So, why would you want to leave trash in your colon for a week? People should poop no less than once per day, some people even poop after every meal!

If you are experiencing the opposite issue and are having too many bowel movements per day, that is another issue. Quick side trip. If you start eating healthier and cut out dairy and grains, most intestinal stuff starts to get better. We will talk about Irritable Bowel and Leaky Gut in the Restore It chapter. That being said, go to my website and get my online program! Yes, now, put down the book and jump online, and do that one thing, then finish reading this chapter.

If you have never been to a chiropractor, or you have had a negative experience, hear me out. Chiropractic care does WAY more than just fix low back or neck pain. In many cases it does a great job at helping both of those conditions, but it actually helps heal your body from the inside, out. When chiropractors adjust the spine, manually or with an instrument, it changes your central nervous system.

There are receptors everywhere on and inside your joints. When the chiropractor adjusts you and stimulates those receptors, it travels through your spinal column to your brain. Your brain receives that information and sends back other information back down to the joint, muscles and other nerves in the surrounding area. If that nerve also happens to go to one of your organs, like your lungs or liver, those organs also receive information when a joint is adjusted. It's like a checkup from the brain via the adjustment. Then, there is also communication from that organ back to the brain and so on... This new communication from the spine to the rest of your body will help put things back in order from the nervous system perspective.

If you think about it, your brain is like the operating system for your communication, the spinal nerves are like the access to the apps like muscles, organs, glands. So, when we adjust the spine it is like an update for the operating system and the apps. Move your spine, it's good for you.

Sleep

Okay, I'm guilty. I've been known to say, "I'll sleep when I'm dead" and "Life is too short to be caught sleeping". AND, I paid dearly for it. Not sleeping after having my children contributed to my post-partum depression and adrenal fatigue. Now lack of sleep can be responsible for much crabbiness in my life. My kids know, mom needs her sleep.

Lack of sleep is at least partially responsible for many chronic diseases. Heart disease, diabetes, high blood pressure, brain fog, immune disorders, adrenal fatigue, infertility and hormone imbalance to name a few. If you have trouble sleeping, these are my top 6 Sleep Hygiene practices.

1. Find and stick to your bedtime. Pick your time. You need 6-8 hours of good sleep every night. Hint: The sleep you get before midnight is actually deeper. The old adage of early to bed, early to rise is true!

2. About an hour before bedtime, make some chamomile tea. Turn off ALL screens, turn down all the lights in your house, light a couple candles. Lavender is relaxing, use a good essential oil like dōTERRA.

3. Do not watch the late news or other stress inducing programs. Violence of any kind is seen by the mind as real. This is a stress, even if you don't find it stressful.

4. Blackout curtains, are an absolute must for any of you all that are unfortunate enough to be working the night shift. If you are on the night shift, keeping your regular sleep hours is crucial to your long-term health. Do not skip sleeping ever! 6 hours minimum!

5. Relaxing music is fine. I have used relaxing guided meditation for years as a sleep aid during stressful times.

6. Napping is fine before 2pm. But, it's not a sleep-a-thon. Only nap 20-30 minutes maximum, any long than this and you will be interrupting sleep later.

To those of you who like some quiet time after the kids go to bed: Consider this. If getting up in the morning is still challenging, and you're falling asleep on the couch at 8pm anyway, first, you are tired! Second, you may be suffering from adrenal fatigue. We will cover this later, suffice to say, do not stay up and wait for the second wind. The dishes, laundry, housekeeping, etc. that you do at night needs to wait. If you go to bed earlier, you will be able to get up earlier, then you can accomplish that stuff in the morning with a clear head and a little more energy. Plus, you will eventually love the peace and quiet when everyone is sleeping, and you are puttering around the house. I know, I hear you saying, "I am NOT a morning person" (emphatic and with whining).

I wasn't a morning person either. However, when I had kids, I figured out that my adrenals were dying and if I didn't get more sleep, I was soon going to be really sick. So, I started going to bed earlier. I found I was able to get up and nurse at around 4am then stay up. That became a pattern for me. I learned that after I got Cooper back to sleep, I would have time to do the dishes, journal, read, have a little time to myself, go to the gym, and be back before the rest of the house got going. That is how this book is being written, in part. I go to bed around 9:30p, get up between 4-5am. YES, some mornings I sleep in till 6 - I allow my body to get the rest it needs. It's a habit and can be changed with an attitude adjustment.

It took time to get used to the new schedule. It will take you time. Anytime we start something new, it feels weird and it is hard. UGH! That **P**rocess thing again. You have to let your body heal, and sleep is part of that healing. Rest and repair. Our bodies are repaired at night. No sleep, or poor sleep, poor repair.

Think and Feel

What is going on in your head? Have you listened to yourself lately? Is it so noisy in your head you can't think? Is the brain fog so thick you are lucky to make it through the day without totally screwing up your life? Or forgetting your youngest at school? Or making it halfway home from Target and you get a text from your child asking where you are, and you realize they are still at Target?

I say some of that in jest, but seriously, what is happening in your head? Do you have the focus and concentration you need? Do you tell yourself what a looser you are? or how fat your butt probably looks? or that you are lazy? What ARE you telling yourself, about yourself? What thoughts spin in your head all day long? Is this really how you want to spend your precious brain energy and your one and only chance at life??

What I am about to tell you may not be something you have ever heard before. ou may choose to believe it or not.

You CAN control what goes on in your head.

There it is. Such a simple sentence and truth. You have 100% control of the thoughts you think and what you choose to believe about yourself. You can change the way you think and what you think. Will it take time?? YES! Will it require constant attention to what IS going on up there? YES!! Will it be worth the months of shushing the noise and reprogramming the voices? YES!! That is how this book was finally written. I had enough of the BS about how I didn't know enough and didn't have anything to say... I was fed up with listening to those voices. Methodically, I started changing what was said. I would catch myself tripping over the old words and put in the new ones. It took time and tears. Clearly, I made it to the other side. If it can happen to write a book, it can happen about weight, career changes or finances or anything else you tell yourself.

So, how did all that crap start in your head? Well, when we are born, we have adults with preformed belief systems raising us. We are submerged into the family environment. We basically believe what we are told. Oh sure, there is rebellion as a teen, and twenty something, but most of our self-esteem and personality is set by the age 6-10, depending on what expert you read.

If you do not know why you feel so bad about yourself, consider the following reasons:

1. Lack of support and approval from your parents and authority figures. Mothers, Fathers, Teachers, Preachers or a reasonable facsimile of any or all of these. Again, this may lead to feelings of inadequacy.

2. Bullying without support from your parents or with overprotective parents. You may actually believe what the bully said about you and you may believe it is okay to be mistreated by other humans. With too much or not enough support, you may not have the necessary skills to stand up for your own beliefs and for yourself. This creates shame. Shame creates blame and anger. This blame and anger can turn inward and create depression and anxiety, or outward and become a combative personality. It is NOT okay!

3. Difficulty with school work may have left you feeling less than adequate. School is not the only form of education in this life, nor does it determine your level of success. Sir Richard Branson barely graduated High School and is one of the richest men on the planet.

4. Social media, news, friends, etc. or any other form of comparison. Comparison causes us to devalue our uniqueness.

This is where **A** - ASK, comes into play. Consider this: If you need help fixing your car, refrigerator, plumbing etc., do you ask for help? Of course you do, especially if your car won't run or your toilet doesn't flush. So, does it make sense to ask for help for yourself?

I have had many coaches and was blessed to find an awesome CBT (cognitive behavioral therapy) therapist that helped me put my kids and I in a better place after I divorced their dad. My EX and I actually get along better now because of some of the skills I learned. I am also more in tune with my intuition and take control of my own emotions. Cognitive Behavioral Therapy is based in the belief that you can change your life by changing your thoughts. This is part of the Positive Psychology movement. This places the changes in your control. Is it easy? No. Is it fast? No. Is it a skill that can be acquired and get easier over time? Yes. It takes practice.

First, some basics about beliefs. We are not aware of these things influencing the way we act and move, the way we make decisions and choices in our life. Some of these beliefs were taught to us as kids and do not serve us as adults. These are known as Limiting Beliefs. Our beliefs are in the subconscious. These antiquated beliefs and belief systems must be acknowledged and changed. Keeping these Limiting Beliefs in mind, we must reprogram our subconscious.

In order to change the underlying belief systems, you have to get in touch with what is going on in the background. Getting still, having some silence is one way to hear what your subconscious is telling you. This is really uncomfortable for some people.

Paying attention to your "gut feelings" or intuition is another way to think about it. Here's the thing, we are so addicted to our busyness and think so many things are important, when they are not, we have lost touch with our intuition. Some of what your intuition has been telling you, you may not know about because you have ignored the signals for so long. You don't know how to face the truth if you <u>have</u> paid attention or just plain don't want to face the truth because it looks too hard and is out of sync with what you think others may want. Your life is your life. What other want is not part of this conversation right now. You may have faced some of your truths, but you are unsure of how to change any of it. Before you stop reading out of overwhelm, read this story.

> I have tried to write this book three other times. But, each time I let something stand in my way. I thought I had too many other things to do and couldn't find time. I thought my business was too big and I didn't have time.

Then I thought I didn't like the way the drafts read. The work didn't sound like me.

Then, I had a coach get to the heart of the matter. It took months. I was afraid of three things. 1. Not pleasing myself. I was afraid it would fail, and I would be a failure. 2. Not pleasing every reader and 3. People wouldn't like me personally. I wouldn't slow down. I was afraid to see what I might find out about myself. That, maybe I was the cause of my failure. Then, I wouldn't be able to blame outside forces for my own behavior. Everything I told myself seemed legit, right?

What I finally realized was the people pleasing, be nice, messages I grew up with, in my subconscious were holding me back. You know that voice that says, "if you can't say something nice, don't say anything"? Yeah, that was holding me back. That is deep in the subconscious. But if I had not gotten still and been honest with myself, I never would have been able to face it down and shift that thought. The thing is, once I got it, I started writing and most of it got positive reviews. How I am going to get this book published is still a mystery. But, I am writing and moving forward.

I knew if I was going to tell the truth, wouldn't be able to always be "nice". Sometimes, the truth isn't nice and doesn't come out nice. What I realized was, that the people reading it would make that decision themselves. That didn't change the truth or me. It was not a reflection on me. It is their own reaction. They chose it. Two people can watch the same movie and have opposing opinions. That doesn't change the movie maker or the honesty of the movie.

Another true story. I have a girlfriend who met a guy. They started dating. Over time she developed stomach issues. She had stomach pain, vomiting, diarrhea - the works. The doctors told her she had Irritable Bowel

Syndrome and she would just have to live with it. They married. Her stomach issues got worse. She ended up with her appendix and gallbladder being removed. She still had the same issues.

Oh, did I tell you that her husband and her fought several times a week, since they started dating. Their relationship was less than harmonious. He played a lot of sports and would stay out with the guys. He was faithful, said he loved her. When she was growing up, her dad was never home. She thought that was the way marriage should look. She did not want to know there were other options. She ignored her intuition, advice from friends and family and remained

Eventually after 10 years of marriage, she finally gave him an ultimatum, he chose sports and they divorced. Her stomach problems went away.

So, if you don't want to hear any more, that is fine. I know I have said the truth and you may not able to process this right now. Our beliefs about the way things are supposed to be, are not always evident. Our beliefs shape our lives and come from our subconscious that may or may not be in tune with what we need in our adult life. Get in touch with what is your own truth.

Here are some tips to digging into your subconscious, listen to your limiting beliefs, find your intuition again and start listening what your body and heart is telling you. IT can be really scary, but none of it will kill you. People go through all kinds of hardships, mentally, emotionally, physically. They endure all kinds of pain because they refuse to listen to their intuition. Once you start hearing heart again, there may be some new pain. Then it's up to you to decide. What are you going to do? Once you know that life isn't what you want, you can stay in your situation, and make the best of it, or you can change it. Try these techniques.

1. Get still. Really look at what you are doing with your time. If it is not essential to life, like food water, clothing or shelter, it can probably wait. No, I am not talking about purchasing you 200th pair of shoes. That can wait or become your reward for taking some time getting to know yourself again.

2. Journal. It doesn't have to be neat, no one has to read it. You can throw away the paper if you don't want someone to read it. Lock the document on your phone or computer. Put it in a personal safe. Just write whatever is coming to your mind. Even if it doesn't make sense. Just write stream of consciousness. Literally, pick a thought and write it

down, pick another and write it down and so on. Give yourself at least 10 minutes. There is a great app for this called the Five Minute Journal.

3. Have gratitude. This is a practice. It works great for anxiety. Anxiety is partially caused by creating negative stories about what MIGHT happen. Anxiety is created by telling yourself stories about the future. Depression is telling yourself stories about the "what could have beens" of the past. Gratitude brings you back to the present and reminds you there are good things that deserve your attention.

4. Pay attention to what your body is telling you. The nudge in your belly, the lump in your throat, that feeling behind your eyes when you see what you want are all clues to your intuition. Your body will tell you when something is right or wrong for you. Your body will also tell you that you have choices you may not have seen before now. Pay attention to your body.

5. Pay attention when you find yourself in a similar situation more than once. You always pick the same kind of guy or girl. You have the same fight with your best friend. There are patterns in our life that we respond to the same way, every time, and then we are unhappy with the results. Look for those patterns and look at what belief you are hanging onto that may not be beneficial to you as an adult. Are you afraid? What is your response or

reaction in these scenarios? What if you changed the way you have these fights or discussions. What if you asked questions instead of reacting irrationally?

6. Meditation and prayer. This is part of getting still. During meditation and prayer, your brain waves actually change and allow you access to deeper parts of your brain and consciousness. There are many ways. I love guided meditations. See my website for my faves.

The Think and Feel piece of Clean It Up will be a lifelong journey. As you learn more about yourself, you will shift your perspective of the world and your life. It's fascinating, challenging, sad and happy all at the same time. And totally worth the effort.

How did I get sick in the first place?

Next to "I feel like crap" the comment I hear most often is "how did I get this way"? The answer is easy and complicated. I'm going to make it as simple as possible.

The first thing to know is your body doesn't forget all the illnesses, medications/toxins, lack of or excessive exercise or sleep, negative situations or people in your life, poor food choices, etc. To establish how you got this way, take a closer look at your health history. Ask yourself the following questions:

1. Breast fed or bottle fed? This makes a difference. Among the plethora of benefits to breast feeding, the beneficial bacteria that grow with breast milk are higher in number and greater in beneficial species than those that grow with formula. This can change digestion and nutrient assimilation. This means you may not be getting the nutrition you need.

2. Were you sick as a kid? ear infections? Tonsillitis? Strep throat? Pneumonia? Allergies? Stomach aches?

3. Did you have more than five rounds of antibiotics as a kid?

4. Teen illnesses? Acne? Hormone/PMS/Bad periods? Mono? Poor sleep habits? Poor eating habits?

5. College and beyond. Alcohol use, more than 5 drinks/beer/wine per week?

6. Other medications? Birth Control Pills? For Acne? For Allergies?

7. Exercise? Excessive or non-existent? Sports? Injuries?

8. Do you drink enough water?

9. How much caffeine do you consume in a day?

10. Trauma? Emotional? Physical? Parents divorced? Moving multiple times? Molested?

When you look at all the potential things that happened to your body, you begin to understand that at some point, something is going to break down. Layer these life events, choices and habits on top of your genetics and you manifest some kind of illness. This is a different view than what you probably think about as your "health". As I stated in the beginning chapters, we are not predestined by our genetics. We know that genetics only play a 10-30% role in the majority of our typical chronic diseases. Since that is true, and we know we have to start to clean it up first.

So, CLEAN IT UP! Clean up the CRAP! Eat, Drink, Move, Sleep Think and Feel is our foundation. We cannot supplement over a bad diet. Yes, it is a Process and NO! Perfectionism is not welcome here. The perfectionist behavior is all about shame. We do not have to do this Cleaning perfectly as it too is a Process... CRAP! Now, the harder work begins. We have to Restore It.

Chapter 5: R: Restore Function
Deep Cellular Change is made here

We are going to go through five pieces of the Restore It phase. Please understand, you may not need to go through every single part of these protocols. I can assure you, that most of you will need the Gut Healing protocol. Our American lifestyle has trashed our stomach and intestines. The next section will explain how all the parts are interrelated. The end of the chapter will detail each protocol and give you all the resources you need to Do It Yourself - Functional Medicine! My goal is to help more people by explaining everything you need to know in an easy to understand format, then detail the steps you need to take control of your health, and frankly, your life. Welcome to DIY-FM.

Is Leaky Gut a Thing?
Yes, it is a thing. It is called many things, in the scientific literature it is known as impaired intestinal

permeability. Dysbiosis or Leaky Gut results from all the trauma you just discovered. All of the poor choices, life events, and habits cause the intestinal lining to start to break down. It is designed to keep out undigested food particles, bacteria, virus, toxins and yeast. However, as time moves forward, and poor choices and habits continue, the lining becomes less picky about what it allows into the body. This is known as increased intestinal permeability or Leaky Gut. Over time, the junk that leaks in, begins turning on your immune system which is located just outside the lining. Your immune system basically gets upset with you and turns against you creating allergies, asthma, joint pain, fibromyalgia, bloating, hormonal hell, adrenal fatigue, thyroid issues, autoimmune diseases like rheumatoid and lupus, and that is just the beginning.

So, YES, Leaky Gut is a thing and it literally effects all of you. Real health begins and ends in the gut.

Gut Healing

We have to restore the gut first. You can take lots of supplements to decrease symptoms. Sure, you can start on adrenal formulas, and immune building and liver detoxes and cleanses, but until the gut is really healed, you will be wasting your money, in my opinion. Putting tons supplements into a Leaky Gut is also a waste, especially if you are having gut symptoms already.

A quick word about supplements. Not all are created equal. Professional brands are more expensive because they guarantee that what is in the bottle is on the label, and if it's on the label, it's in the bottle. There are plenty of reports about over the counter supplements not even containing the main ingredients that were listed on the label. If a supplement doesn't work, you have wasted your money. I have created a Basic and Comprehensive supplement protocol for each Restore It program. Okay, onward!

There are 4 main processes that have to be restored:

1. Digestion and Assimilation. This refers to how your food is broken down into its component parts.

    1.1. Proteins, like meat, beans, tofu, are made of amino acids. When the food reaches the stomach, Hydrochloric acid, HCl, is necessary in appropriate quantities to start breaking down proteins and turn on other enzymes needed to complete protein digestion and help your body make B-12. The proteins need to be fully broken down into their component parts, called amino acids, or your body cannot absorb and use, or assimilate, the amino acids to make muscle tissue and enzymes. Enzymes help to make other reactions happen throughout your body and keep it running. When proteins are not being broken down properly, muscle tissue and detoxification really suffer.

1.2. Fats also need to be digested and broken down to become parts of cell structure and other fat containing molecules. Your Liver and Gallbladder are responsible for the breakdown and processing of fats. Your liver makes bile. Bile is stored in the gallbladder until you eat. When you eat, the gallbladder is signaled by the brain to dump its contents into the small intestine, where it helps fat become more absorbable. If you no longer have a gallbladder, you may not produce enough bile to breakdown the fat properly. This can lead to feeling full all the time, nausea, vomiting, and greasy, foul-smelling stools. Long term effects of the inability to digest fats included vitamin A, D, E, K deficiencies, immune and inflammatory disorders, cholesterol issues, hormonal imbalance. Dehydration is also common. When cells are inflamed and not made of good ingredients, they also get leaky, and your body doesn't hold water inside the cells as it should. A Bio-Impedance analysis can be done in my office to determine the level of dehydration, and how much water in inside your cells vs outside your cells.

1.3. Carbohydrates are broken down primarily for energy. But, if they are not digested properly, can lead to bloating and gas. Digestion starts in the mouth with an enzyme called alpha amylase. This starts breaking down carbs first thing. Your mom always said to chew your food, your stomach doesn't have teeth.

1.4. As I mentioned earlier, when the food reaches the stomach, Hydrochloric acid, HCl, is necessary in appropriate quantities to start breaking down proteins and turn on other enzymes needed to complete protein digestion and help your body make B-12. Here's what you don't know and probably have learned the exact opposite. When there is a lack of stomach acid, GERD or reflux, also known as heartburn results. I know, this concept is completely contrary to what you have been told about heartburn. By this point in the book you shouldn't be surprised that I have a different take on what the media and Pharma has been selling you for the last 40 years. But, as you have cleaned up your diet, some of your heartburn should have gone away anyway. Taking out the heavy carbs, slow down to eat, you cannot digest your food if your body thinks you are running away from danger all the time. As you allow your body to heal these symptoms will start to decrease.

This is where a supplement can really help. My favorite digestive enzyme formula, which contains HCl, is by OrthoMolecular, called Digestzyme and Pure Encapsulations Digestive Enzymes Ultra with HCl. If you have ulcers, go easy on this one, and preferably, start

Mucosagen for at least two weeks. Also, from OrthoMolecular, it helps your body recreate the mucus lining of your stomach and allowing it to heal. The other way to go is to use Spectrazyme Complete from Metagenics and add Spectrazyme Metagest for the HCl separately. You have to get both of these supplements through a health practitioner. More instructions and you have access to some of my professional brands are available through my website, DrKrisSargent.com.

1.5. Impaired Intestinal Permeability Ah yes, Leaky Gut. Healing MUST begin here. You can Clean It Up, then Restore It starts here. If you haven't done an actual gut healing protocol while eating clean, you have missed 50-75% of the healing. There are several highly effective substances like specific amino acids, herbs and vitamins, which have been shown to restore the gut lining. If you have a history of ulcers and reflux, as I mentioned above, Mucosagen and/or Glutagenics will help start the healing. Then, a product like InflammaCore or UltraInflamX will really help the healing process along. Both of these products are anti-inflammatory powders, based in rice and pea protein, with bio-available Turmeric and L-glutamine to heal the "Leaky". You can put them a smoothie with almond or coconut milk and 1/2 cup of berries, and VOILA! You have breakfast, lunch or a snack. In the comprehensive plan, I have added GlutaShield or Glutagenics. This gives you a higher dose of L-Glutamine along with Probiotic 225 (225 BILLION) organisms. You can put all three of these products in a smoothie. Start slow with the InflammaCore/UltraInflamX. Start with half a scoop for 2-3days, one scoop for 2-3 days and then two scoops, onward. You may not be able to take the entire two scoops. Two to eight weeks into the process you may start to feel horrible. Your body is shifting to a more anti-inflammatory state and you are detoxing. You are healing and some of the unfriendly bacteria, in your gut are dying. You can imagine the carnage! These unfriendly bacteria have had years of sugar and processed food and now they are dying, leaving their own toxins and dead carcasses everywhere. No worries, your body will Clean It Up in a few days with all the good nutrition and this will pass. Literally, expect to be pooping regularly. More on elimination below. You can find more information about detoxing on my website and YouTube channel.

2. Bug Balance. One of the coolest facts about the body is we house 100 TRILLION organisms in our guts. WOW! Yes, there are more bacteria and yeast in your intestines than cells in your body. There are friendly ones and unfriendly ones. With years of processed foods and sugar and all the other life events, habits and choices, the unfriendly ones will

reign, like a bad gang. It is important to get these dudes back under control. The unfriendly bacteria and yeast will prevent hormones from being detoxed properly, create their own toxins, prevent vitamins from being made and cause chronic infections. These unfriendly bacteria, viruses and yeasts also ignite your immune system causing you to feel drained. These bad gang members can potentially be the beginning of an auto-immune disorder if left unchecked for years. Did you hear that!! It is really important to get your gut healed so your immune system can heal!

An aside about unfriendly yeast. The most prevalent, illusive and frustrating yeast to control is called Candida. It may be on the loose in your body. It doesn't just set up house in your guts though, chronic sinus issues, vaginal infections, and throat infections are often caused by yeast. When we are under stress, make poor life choices, have negative life events and habits, our body makes different chemistry to deal with the stress. It is basically compensating for being chased by a Bengal tiger all the time, as I mentioned before. Long term stressors also change the type of bacteria and yeast that set up house in our guts, sinuses and vaginas. You have taken the first step to getting this under control by Cleaning It Up and using this Gut Healing Protocol. We will take more measures in the not too distant future. Let's get some nutrition and healing started, the number of unfriendly bugs will decrease by taking these steps. Rest assured, we will get some yeast killing herbs on those left over stubborn Candida and other bacteria, if necessary.

The friendly bacteria help us digest our food, feed the cells of our intestine, and make vitamins that help our body do what it needs to do at the cellular level. After all, we are made up of trillions of cells, if the cells aren't able to do their job, what happens to the body as a whole? We need to feed these guys a friendly environment, so they can take over the turf from the bad bugs. Changing your diet, will help immensely. You can change the bugs in as little as 3 days! Getting a handle on as many of the previously mentioned stressors from the Clean It Up chapter as possible will make a positive shift in the Bug Balance. Now you have an understanding about why these are so important to our health and how they can mess with your health if there is an imbalance.

3. Elimination You MUST poop every day. Period. The end... no other way. Even if you have never pooped every day, we have to get you pooping. The first step is changing the type of food and personal water consumption. Once those two habits are in place, make sure you have time every morning to poop, assuming you are a morning pooper. DO

NOT suppress the urge to poop until a more convenient time. That will ultimately lead to constipation. Also, running from that tiger right out of the gate in the morning, isn't really the way to poop either. Yes, warm beverages like water with lemon will help. Coffee or tea may help because the caffeine plus the warmth, starts the intestines moving. That being said, caffeine has some plusses and minuses that need to be considered. Caffeinated beverages ultimately dehydrate the body and cause stress on blood sugar maintenance, the adrenals and liver detoxification. Your functional medicine doctor should help you figure out whether caffeine is a good alternative for you. A couple immediate recommendations to support colon cleansing include using what I call the Constipation Cocktail. Magnesium Citrate, Vitamin C and High Potency Omega 3 Fish Oil (look at the label, add EPA+DHA>1000). How to use the Constipation Cocktail:

1. Day 1: 100mg of Magnesium citrate plus 2000mg of Vitamin C and 2 Fish Oil, in the evening before bed.

2. If you do not poop in the morning then start to increase the Magnesium and Vitamin C. Day 2: 200mg Mg Citrate, 3000mg Vitamin C, 2 Fish Oil - still evening before bed

3. If still no poop: Day 3: 300 mg Mg Citrate, 4000 Vitamin C, 2 Fish oil

4. Continue to increase if no poop: 400mg Mg Citrate; 4000mg Vitamin C, 2 Fish oil

5. Day 5: If you are not pooping: Double everything - I would wait for a weekend to try this. 800mg Mg Citrate; 8000mg Vitamin C and Fish oil. If this protocol does not work, I use a product that contains Cape Aloe. This is a specific type of aloe, not typical Aloe Vera. The product I use in my practice is Super Aloe 250 and Super Aloe 450 from OrthoMolecular, available on my FullScript site.

Detoxification is also part of elimination. This takes place in your liver and kidneys, primarily. We take in so many toxins and because we have a liver and kidneys, we usually don't know anything about it. These amazing organs take potential poisons and turn them into something water soluble, so these nasty substances can be eliminated from your body. It's like taking out the trash. When we have eaten CRAP, and our body doesn't have the nutrients you need to accomplish detoxification, symptoms can arise. The symptoms may include nausea, foggy brain, hormone disruptions, acne, fatigue, migraines, joint and muscle pain, and more. Starting the with The Clean It Up program, will improve detoxification, just getting better food in your body will give it the new nutrients it needs to do the detox job. Let me say this very plainly, our bodies need the nutrients in vegetables and fruits to detox. These help create what is known as antioxidants. Antioxidants are involved in detox and slow the aging process. We will go through this in more detail when I outline the Liver Detox and Regeneration program.

Before I move on, you will need to discover where you are with your healing program. You can go on my website and click on Health Evaluation link to get a free assessment or you can go by the general guidelines. My online class goes over this in detail.

Basic Gut Healing Protocol

If you have been on a gluten free and dairy free diet, a Candida diet, GAPS, FODMAP etc. for more than 3 months and have been 90% compliant with it (perfectionism is NOT welcome here), shift to RENEW diet, found on my website. The following supplements can be found at metagenics.com or FullScript link on my website www.DrKrisSargent.com:

Basic Bundle: UltraInflamX/InflammaCore, Probiotic with over 200 billion CFU's, Digestive enzyme like Spectrazyme Complete or Digestzyme, High potency natural Multivitamin like AlphaBase or PhytoMulti and Vitamin D3.

The UIX can be made into a smoothie w 1/2 cup berries and 6 ounces of unsweetened almond or coconut milk and ice.

If you are healing, weight loss may or may not happen at this point. However, calories do count.

Comprehensive Gut Healing Protocol

Adding a couple more supplements to encourage faster healing, and give the body more of the healing ingredients, I add Glutagenics or GlutaShield. One scoop of either, added to the smoothie above, will add 4 more grams of L-Glutamine. L-Glutamine is an amino acid which helps heal the gut.

Gut healing takes time, 2-6 months from my experience. How do you know when you are healed? Take the Health Evaluation again. See where your numbers improved. Look at your life. Take a self-inventory of what has changed in your health. Energy? Sleep? Moods? Hormones? Sinuses? Gut pain, bloating?

Return to my website and take your Health Assessment again. At this point, some specific nutrition will be needed. It depends on who you are, your personal history and ability to heal. Your Immune system, Liver or Adrenals/Hormones, may still be an issue. Energy, mood swings, sensitivity to foods, still have some rumbly guts? Stay on the Gut Healing protocol. After the first month, you can drop the Probiotic 225 and start a good probiotic from Metagenics, like UltraFlora Balance or Probiotic 100 from OrthoMolecular.

Immune Reboot

As your gut starts healing you will notice your inflammation going down. You will have less pain, less bloating and feel less swollen, in general. Your immune system is responding by decreasing the overall level of inflammation. The immune system is highly complex, so, as usual, I will do my best to break it down into simpler parts.

Without our immune system we would not make it very long in this world. The onslaught of bacteria, viruses and fungi that are around to assault us is staggering. Part of our immune system is designed to defend our body. Another part of the immune system is designed to repair our body. This works to repair the everyday wear and tear, regenerating our hair, skin, nails, liver cells, red and white blood cells, just to name a few. It also repairs the body when it has gotten sick or injured. Our body can heal itself. You have seen it happen since you were a kid. Scraped you knee when you fell off your bike? It was gone in a matter of a few days. Bigger injuries take more time. Lifetime injuries take a longer time.

There are many things that can happen when our immune systems get whacked out by our leaky gut. When there is damage to the lining of your intestine, as in Leaky Gut, "Inflammation" is the process that generally starts healing the body. It goes crazy and doesn't shut off when it is bombarded with more damaging insults.

The food we eat, or don't eat, carries messages to our body. Those messages can be healing or harmful. The foods most commonly associated with inflammatory messages are wheat, barley and rye (gluten containing grains), gluten, dairy, eggs, soy, and sugar (all forms in greater than a couple teaspoons per day including honey, maple syrup, agave, coconut, etc.), processed foods in boxes or bags (chips, pasta, bread, crackers, cookies etc.). Yes, your food talks to your body. Messages may be healing or hurtful, you chose that message every time you eat.

When the body is constantly bombarded with these negative messages. The inflammation continues to rise. Typically, if we have pain or stiffness or a headache, we will take an aspirin or ibuprofen. Once in a while, this is fine. However, continued daily use over time, increases Leaky Gut by further breaking down the intestinal lining. You may have less pain, but, the damage is still happening. It is at this point when our immune system gets so pissed off it starts making antibodies to our own body parts. This is known as auto-immunity and is part of the Root Cause of auto-immune disorders.

Antibodies are generally good things that are like heat seeking missiles for invaders like bacteria or viruses. The antibodies help other cells in your immune system recognize the invaders as foreign, so those cells can destroy the invader. Think of antibodies like a flag, marking a spot. The immune cells see the flag and now knows exactly where to go and what to kill. However, when the immune system is on high alert for a long period of time, because of poor lifestyle habits we have discussed throughout this book, your immune system starts making antibodies to your own parts. This is what we call "Auto" (meaning self) immune diseases. There are hundreds of autoimmune diseases. Any organ, gland, or tissue can have an antibody created against it. That means joint tissue of rheumatoid, soft tissue, like connective tissue of Sjogren's, Hashimoto's or Graves of the thyroid, Multiple Sclerosis in the brain etc., all auto-immune disorders have the same origin - an immune system gone crazy!

The destruction that our immune system may create is heart-breaking for me. Especially since I know that a shift in diet and lifestyle would potentially put it in remission, I have seeing happen in thousands of cases.

Until the foods are gone, for about 90 days or more, the inflammation doesn't go away. Please plan for healing to take time. Last time I checked, magic wands and magic pills were permanently backordered on Amazon! The biological drugs offered by the medical system are not designed to be used for a lifetime, so what are you going to do? If your health issues are lifestyle based, all the drugs and supplements in the world are not going to help you in the long run.

Get the foundation of your health right. Clean up your lifestyle then add any one of the natural anti-inflammatories that will help support inflammation and modify your immune response.

Liver Detoxification and Regeneration

The liver and kidneys, along with the small and large intestines (your guts) are responsible for assimilation of foods, drinks into your body and getting the toxins out of your body. These organs transform what you eat and drink into energy, muscles, blood cells, your immune cells and system, bone, hormones, neurotransmitters, and all of your communication molecules and new body pieces that are worn out and need replacing. Your cell structure is made and replaced all the time. We tend to think of our body as something stable, our heart, lungs, liver, intestines, but the cells of each body part and system is very dynamic, breaking down and/or building up all the time. Every time you eat something, you can either create positive or negative reactions in your body. We need macronutrients such as protein, carbohydrates and fats to make a healthy body. Certain body types may need more or less of any one macronutrient.

Our body also requires micronutrients such as vitamins and minerals. Our food contains many of the vitamins and minerals we need. Because of the tremendous stresses in our "typical" American lifestyle, I also believe good quality supplementation is mandatory to heal and stay healthy. The liver requires a ton of these macro and micronutrients to do its job.

There are two reasons I do not think liver detoxification plans are okay until the gut is healed. First, let's say you are going to move some junk from your basement to your garage. But when you get to the garage it is full. The full garage represents a gut that has not been working properly. There is no place

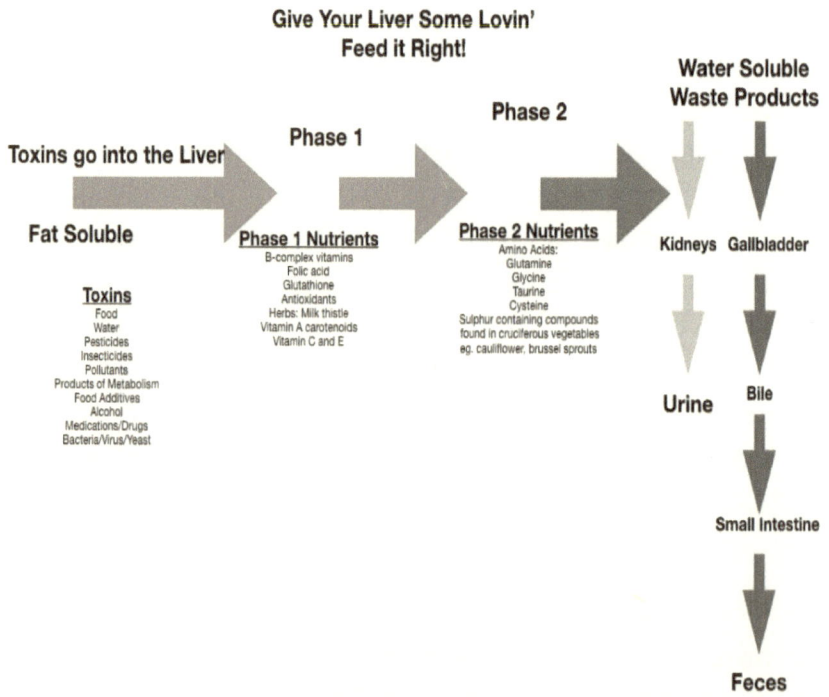

to put the stuff from the basement. You have to clean out the garage - the Gut - before you dump the contents of your basement - the Liver - into your gut. So, gut healing first. Many times, cleaning up and healing your gut, will help your liver do its job naturally. If you are still experiencing gallbladder issues, headaches, itchy skin, hives and rashes you will need deeper liver cleansing.

Second, if your gut is that much of a mess, and liver detoxification needs a lot of extra nutrients, how are the nutrients going to get in through the mess?

So, in Functional Medicine, liver function improvement usually follows improvements in the gut function. Yes, everyone is different, and it doesn't mean that both aren't going to happen at the same time anyway. But, to compartmentalize each process seems to make sense for descriptive purposes.

THIS IS AN IMPORTANT POINT! Please remember that everything you are doing to heal your gut... is healing your whole body! Adrenals benefit from keeping your blood sugar even. Your liver benefits from having more nutrients to detox the junk with, your hormones can be happier because insulin and cortisol are no longer running the show (both are very stressful for your body when not controlled). You are doing most of the right stuff already. When we discuss liver detox, we are really talking about improving liver function, so your body can be more efficient at doing all of its jobs.

Please know, these processes take very specific nutrients. And a LOT of them. Detoxification is no simple system. So, lets discover how it works.

The liver and kidneys take in everything you ingest and breathe. For our purposes think food and toxins. Remember toxins are in your food, in the air you breathe, in the water you drink in the meds you take, they are everywhere. Even eating perfectly organic, grass fed, raised in bubble food doesn't exempt you from having toxins in your system.

So, let's start with proteins. The proteins you eat get broken down to amino acids, by peptidases and HCl, hydrochloric acid in your stomach. The food moves out of the stomach and are absorbed through the small intestines. These amino acids are shunted to every cell in your body to make enzymes, muscle cells, cell structural components, hormones, neurotransmitters, and more! This is why proper stomach function is so critical for good health. Without proper digestion your body cannot get what it needs for new parts!

Protein plays a crucial role in water balance of the body. Albumin is a protein made by the liver, Albumin is a shuttle for hormones and other cell communicators, and minerals. Albumin also important for that water balance and can cause edema and swelling when things are out of balance. Other proteins like Sex Hormone Binding Globulin and Thyroxine Binding Globulin, to name a couple, are important for shuttling estrogen, testosterone and thyroid hormone. And this is just the tip of the iceberg. Amino acids make up the components of the liver enzymes that are responsible for the detoxification process.

Carbohydrates sources are fruits and vegetables, preferentially for our purposes. Complex carbohydrates, those with higher carbohydrate concentration per mouthful, include some fruits, bananas/grapes, grains and starchy vegetables. These are considered important for energy production because they can be easily broken down into the glucose molecule. Glucose is the easy fuel for our cells. The problem with excess carbohydrate consumption, more than about 20 grams per meal, is that our body will have to store what it cannot fit into our cells. Go back to our blood sugar discussion.

When we eat carbs, like I described before, insulin is released. Insulin tries to get glucose into the cells. When it has done the best it can, excess glucose has to go to the liver to be package up into a molecule called triglycerides. Glucose and triglycerides effect cholesterol production. That is why eating red meat isn't the problem when you have high cholesterol. More than likely, it is the high carb diet. So, the liver is where cholesterol and most other fats are produced.

Fats coming into your body can be inflammatory or anti-inflammatory. It is well established that medium chain triglycerides like coconut oil are beneficial.

Avocados, nuts and seeds are also great sources of healthy fats. Your liver has to make sure you can get those fats into your body. It makes bile, which is stored and concentrated in the gallbladder. Bile gets squirted into the small intestine when food, at the proper pH, passes from the stomach into the small intestine. SEE! The stomach HAS to have the right pH, and the right amount of stomach acid for food to move into the small intestine and signal the brain to contract the gallbladder and stimulate the pancreas to release the rest of the enzymes necessary to break down the food. Everything works together.

A side note about acid blocking drugs and stress. Both of these will decrease stomach acid production. I just told you, the pH of the contents of your stomach is crucial for proper digestive processes. Both cause the body to push undigested food into the small intestine. But, the signals to the gallbladder and pancreas may not fully function. Food goes undigested, you feel bloated, and gassy because the bacteria are now fermenting your food giving off methane and hydrogen gas. If methane is in excess, it can cause constipation, if hydrogen is in excess, you may get diarrhea.

Aside from the assimilation functions of the liver it also must take toxins from your blood and make them into less toxic molecules, so the body can get rid of them, safely. Many toxins are not water soluble, so the liver has to change those toxins from fat soluble to water soluble. Changing toxins to water-soluble molecules is a two-step process. Here is the real piece of information you need, detoxification requires a LOT of nutrients. So, if you have been eating CRAP for a long time, your liver isn't able to be very efficient. Throw CRAP food on top of poor detoxing genetics and you could be a mess. So, give your liver some lovin' and feed it right.

Adrenal Rebuild and Hormonal Balancing

Your adrenals are walnut sized glands on the top of your kidneys. The adrenals are responsible for water and mineral balance, and hormone balance. The adrenals produce cortisol and adrenaline under stressful situations. Cortisol breaks down muscle tissue to feed the brain, along with creating inflammation, and adrenaline raises your heart rate, and shunts blood to the muscles, away from digestion. This is why stress is so destructive. It breaks down muscle tissue and disrupts digestion.

To rebuild your adrenals and start balancing your hormones, the two most important habits you MUST create are a steady blood sugar level and sleep! We have discussed blood glucose levels several times. Eating small frequent meals with protein, vegetables, fat and fiber about 100-200 calories every 3-4 hours will create the need for lower insulin and glucose levels. This leads to less inflammation and stress. Sleep. Your body requires a minimum of 6 hours of uninterrupted sleep every night. Yes, 7-8 hours are better and will help you heal faster.

A couple of symptoms that may remain are that second wind between 8-9 pm and problems with your period or menopause.

You sit down at 7:30-8 and fall asleep, but if you get up and try to go to bed you are awake. What this requires is a few weeks of going to bed early. I know, you have little kids, you are single, your husband doesn't help, lots of reasons not to go to bed. The most common reason I hear is, "that is my winding down time".

I fully understand! AND, you have to figure out whether you feel bad enough to shift?

Is it worth changing a sleep pattern, that IS JUST a habit? You really CAN be a morning person! Do you believe it is something ingrained in a person? No, it's a habit we create over time. If someone told you that your life depended on you becoming a morning person - you would figure it out. So, no excuses, figure it out. We tell ourselves stories about how we hate mornings and love our evening times. That said, if you have time to actually sleep in the morning that is wonderful. Studies have shown that sleep before midnight is actually more restful sleep. So, try going to bed early for a month. YES, a month. You may find you are up early, like even 4 am! And think about it, you were sleeping from midnight until 6am, now you are waking up on your own after sleeping the same 6 hours 10pm - 4am. Instead of cursing the early hour, could you choose to embrace it? Could you get up early and journal, read, meditate or go to the gym? Could you get the laundry started or clean the kitchen?

That is a pattern I established when my kids were little. Actually, I was nursing Cooper, my youngest. He would nurse at 3:30-4 and I would stay up after I get him back to sleep. The house was quiet, I could think, and read, and plan, and journal. It was great. I would go to the gym as soon as it opened, and by 6am I felt like I had accomplished a ton! And no one had even stirred yet. Just try it.

If you continue to have groggy mornings, looking for coffee or other stimulants, then have a hard time settling down in the evening, and are looking for alcohol, you will need to use some herbal adaptogens for a short time.

Herbal adaptogen protocol: I like AdrenAll from OrthoMolecular or Adrenogen or Licorice Plus (not for people with high blood pressure) from Metagenics to help support the adrenals in the morning. Then I like AdreneVive in the late afternoon to help control cortisol. I have also had success with Serenagen from Metagenics. For sleep issues, I like Botanicalm Pm from OrthoMolecular or MetaRelax or TranQ from Metagenics.

A note about coffee and alcohol. Coffee in 8-16 ounce servings first thing in the morning as a ritual is common. Coffee used throughout the day to keep yourself focused and awake is destructive. It forces your adrenals to make adrenaline. This shuts down your digestion and overstimulates your adrenals, causing them to function poorly in the long run. Alcohol used to "take the edge off" is interfering with your sleep patterns and hormones. It screws with your blood sugar and sucks B-complex vitamins out of your body. I am not saying that a couple glasses of wine on the weekend is bad. Just know what you may be causing when you are imbibing more frequently.

For menopause and peri-menopause, alcohol, sugar and caffeine make hot flashes worse and will put hormones out of balance, as well. Your body cannot create hormone balance without proper sleep patterns and drinking wine every evening will interfere with healthy sleep patterns.

Premenstrual Syndrome, Peri-menopause and Menopause

I am going to address certain specific issues later in the book, but since we are talking about hormone balance I thought it would be important to say couple things. First, **PMS** mood swings, low energy, heavy periods, irregular periods, cramping are common.

HOWEVER, they are NOT normal!! Your period should be a non-event. "Oh, look, I'm bleeding." That's it.

You do not have to live with ridiculous periods!! Frankly, my horrible PMS probably helped destroy many relationships in my life and ended up putting me in touch with a great vitamin rep from a little company, at the time, called Metagenics. I am still grateful for that Metagenics rep that taught me about hormone balance, B-complex vitamins, helped me clean up my gut and liver and set my life on a steady pattern of easy periods and introduced me to the world of Functional Medicine and Dr Jeffrey Bland, while I was still in school.

Having my kids at around 40, put my hormones back into a tailspin, and it took me 3 years to regain some semblance of normalcy in my periods. It took my 5 years to regain my immune system control I really understand the time and dedication it takes to a create a clean, steady lifestyle. I had thyroid and adrenal issues coming off both my pregnancies. It took a long time to get things straight again.

T Functional Medicine techniques and practices I am sharing with you are exactly what I did to heal.

Peri-Menopause is a time of shifting hormones. Do not expect every month to be the same. Most women are in need of some help with their progesterone production. When the adrenals make excessive cortisol over time due to stress, the body can lack progesterone. That doesn't mean hormone replacement is the only way to go. There are herbs which can look like progesterone. Chateberry or Vitex is that herb. It proves very useful in straightening out timing issues.

The way we detoxify estrogen, especially after ovulation is also important. I3C from Metagenics or EstroDIM from OrthoMolecular are important supplements to make sure your body is clearing estrogen. When estrogen spikes after ovulation, it creates the symptoms associated with PMS - the bloating, acne, breast tenderness, and then a heavy, painful period. The other part of this story are the inflammatory chemicals produced when we eat like CRAP. Fish oil, omega 3 essential fatty acid balance is important here. You will need high doses of EPA and DHA. At least 2-4 grams per day to help with the pain and get things balanced again.

If you can get your PMS and peri-menopause under control, menopause doesn't have to be too bad. Yes, there are times when hormone replacement is necessary. But herbals can go a long way. Protocols:

PMS:

1. Get your blood sugar even. If you aren't going to eat right, don't bother trying a bunch of other stuff.

2. Chasteberry Plus from Metagenics has been my go to product for decades for irregular periods. Most patients get relief with 1-2 capsules per day.

3. EstroDIM or MetaI3C will help with the bloating, sore boobs, bitchy, bummed out feeling of PMS. Most patients get relief with 1-2 capsules per day.

4. Orenda Otropin and Immune - Otropin helps your pituitary tell your adrenals, ovaries (if you still have them) and your thyroid what to do. Stress and inflammation can interfere with the communication between the pituitary and the other glands. Otropin clears up the communication. Immune helps improve detoxification of hormones, along with improving the immune system overall. Otropin is taken 4 sprays at night under the tongue, then 2 sprays in the morning. Less is more - you may need less of a dose the longer you are on it. If symptoms increase, go to a lower dose. Click on the Orenda Link on my website.

Yes, you can take either or both. Start with one at a time, so you know how it works. Try each one for at least 2 cycles.

Peri-Menopause and Menopause:

1. Blood sugar maintenance is a MUST or don't bother. Sugar, alcohol and caffeine will make all the symptoms worse, decrease their use as much as possible - not perfection!!

2. Try the PMS protocols first

3. Orenda Otropin and Immune. See above description.

WELL! That was a LOT! Restoring function of the body is not for the faint of heart. It can take a long time and can be discouraging. Remember, I have been there! I get it! That takes us through Restoring Function. We have worked our way through the most common areas of dysfunction, explained their root cause and put forth some solutions. Now what?

Chapter 6: A: Action

Which ridiculous do you want?

Which ridiculous do you want? The ridiculousness of your current reality or the ridiculousness of the work you have to put in to change it? Put another way. Life is hard, which "hard" do you want? The "hard" of your current life, OR the "hard" work it takes to change it? To put it a more in your face way, which do you prefer, your current suckiness or your new awesomeness? Crapulous or Fabulous?

This really popped for me! When I really started to assess what was working in my life and what wasn't working, I realized the ridiculous or hard things in my life were all created by MOI! Yep, I created them. UGH! Right?!? That is some hard truth to swallow when personal responsibility is staring you in the face. I created my own sucky situations?? YEP!

I looked at the current reality around my weight and health, my personal relationships, my finances, my kids, and significant other. I asked myself what was working? What needs a tweak? What needs an overhaul? In my life, a couple categories stood out like a sore thumb. Those needed major overhauls! This book is part of my solution. I knew I needed to take a stand for what I believe to be true about healing and true health. I could no longer stand by and watch my great country of the USA get sicker and sicker and fatter and fatter, younger and younger people being effected by CRAP!

Is it hard? Yes, and no. It's hard to know that some people will vehemently object to what I am saying and my truths. But, standing for my truths… I am empowered! And I want to empower you as well.

The results will be amazing! My beliefs are on paper, in audio and video. This is me. I am standing for what I know to be my truth and hopefully you resonate with it. I know the results are not only going to help a bazillion people but will help me too! It will change the world! I asked myself every day, current suckiness or new awesomeness? I choose new awesomeness, new ridiculous, new hard, Fabulous!

So, which ridiculous DO you want? Bluntly, do you want your current reality? Are there parts of your current reality that are ridiculously hard? Your lack of energy and feeling like CRAP every day? Your inability to climb the stairs without being short of breath? What is your current health reality? How is your life being effected by your current health? What would be different if you made a change? Have you taken the Functional Health Reality Check? It's on my website.

OR…

Do you want something different? The "different" will become your new reality. The "different" will feel weird in the beginning. That is the new "ridiculous" you get to feel. The new "hard" is the work of changing. You have to work at change. Even simple tasks like changing the bed, require work. Why would changing a habit be expected to be easy? So, I am going to ask it in a new way, which would you prefer, your current suckiness or your possible awesomeness?

What do you want your health to look like next year at this time? It can be the same, better or worse. What makes the difference? If you continue to do what you are doing, what will your health look like in a year? The same, better or worse? If you decide to shift your lifestyle to what is outlined in this book, what do you think will happen? What will be better? Relationships? Activities? Enjoyment? Digestion? Energy?

Change feels icky, it isn't something you can "see" yourself doing, it isn't "you". All of those things are correct. You created your current reality and you can create a new reality. You have the power!

Is your current health reality a reflection of your current health habits? YES! Your health is the accumulation of everything that has ever happened to your body. Can habits be changed? YES! That is the new ridiculous. The ridiculous work of change vs. the ridiculous of your current reality.

A series of tough questions helped me move forward. Ask yourself the following:

1. The first, most important, and most difficult question...When am I going to start loving myself? So, seriously WHEN is that going to start for you? When am I going to start choosing what is right for me without thinking it's selfish? When am I going to finally DECIDE that your life is valuable? This questioned was posed by one, okay several, of my coaches over a ten-year period. So, no worries if you don't have a lightning bolt experience. AND if you do, let me know about it on my website or Facebook, I love great stories!

2. What is my heart telling me I need to do in my life? STOP and listen to that wee little voice. Feel into that question. Did your heart leap, stomach get bubbly? Here is where you need to be a fan of Horton Hears a Who. In short, Horton was an elephant who saw a little puff ball float by him one day. He swore he heard a voice coming from that puff ball. Turns out there was a whole town, Whoville, on the puff. But, because the other characters in the story couldn't hear the voices because they wouldn't really listen, Horton was tortured and thought to be crazy! We torture ourselves when we don't listen to that little voice. If you haven't paid attention to that little voice in your head or heart for a long time, you may not be able to hear it very well. Journal the thoughts you

wouldn't tell anyone. Journal about what you used to love to do as a kid, or what you used to dream about doing. Journal about the things society says to you about what you want to do. Make a vision board. Check my website I may hold a vision board webinar!

3. What would be improved if I changed my lifestyle? Relationships? My water drinking habit? My time management habits? Or any number of other things I do, most likely, mindlessly, day in and day out. Behavior is just a habit.

4. What is the one habit I can change today to start changing my life? It doesn't have to be a big thing. What if you just drank one more glass of water today? What if I got up 30 minutes earlier to walk? What if I started keeping track of my steps every day, and added 100 steps a day for 30 days? 60 days? 90 days? These small changes over time add up. These are called micro-habits. When you look ahead one year, it seems like forever, but one day? That is doable. Then you do it again.

5. Where will my health be in a year of I do not change anything? Is this what I want? And did I just hear my small voice say, "UGH!" and then I heard it whine like a teenage girl, "but I don't waaannnttt toooo". Did I hear that noise? Okay... this is what you do... Tell it to shut up and sit the F*#@ DOWN! Tell that whiny little voice who is in charge. How does that feel?

6. What am I currently using to distract myself into NOT changing my habits? Um, this is big, do not blow this off. I have been in practice for 25 years as I write this book. Let me tell you, I have heard some of the most elaborate distractions, excuses, and stories people tell themselves about themselves and their lives! Seriously, sometimes I walk out of my office so frustrated because I can see so much that others cannot. Please be honest with yourself.

An executive life coach, friend and my kids' dad says: "An excuse is just a reason with a lie attached". Is everything I am telling myself about my current reality the truth or could I be wrong? Here's the cool part. If you have discovered that maybe, just maybe things could be different, first of all, you don't have to tell anyone; and second, you have all the power to change it! YES, I DO have all the power to change it, after all, I created it in the first place.

Short story. I have a weight loss program that is basically 5 meal replacements and one "regular" meal per day. It is simple. You pick 5 meal replacements out of your supply. And have some 5-7 ounces of lean protein and vegetables once a day. These meal replacements are as simple as a bar or shake and as complicated as cup-a soup or the individual packages of mac and cheese. Literally a meal in 7-8 minutes or less. Perfectly balanced nutritionally, vitamins and minerals, no artificial additives or preservatives, pretty clean. SUPER simple. Makes eating healthy easy. One of my clients is a busy single, mom, getting her kids off to college. Works full-time. She is struggling with her weight and feels like CRAP every day. She barely has the energy to do her normal routine and doesn't make healthy food choices because she is on the run, ENTER my suggestion that she start this program. My meal replacement program solves her time, food, energy and weight issues. She cannot see how it would make her life simpler. She defers until things "settle down". I see both sides, I am non-judgmental. You have to be ready to see your reality for what it is...

Now, what am I missing? Journal about it, think about it, process it with a professional or a really good girlfriend that doesn't let you BS yourself, listen to that wee voice in my head and heart. There are other ways. There are other options. The options may not feel good. OR they may offer the breakthrough I am looking for in my life.

7. Make a list of all the options you have in your life. Even the most absurd options. Yes, even the ones that make no sense whatsoever. Consider every possibility. Keep the list and do not let it overwhelm you. It is just an exercise to see options that you may not have seen before now. If you like one of them, what is the first small step you can take today to get closer to that option?

8. List all the things that will improve when I shift my health. What are some things that I have always wanted to do but cannot because of health reasons? Next step, make a vision board. Tell yourself, I am making this board to make those things concrete in my mind. Ignore the possible ridicule from your spouse, mom, kids and friends. Do it anyway. You cannot change them. You can only change yourself. Those things on that board will become more important than current habits.

That list of things that will change for the better needs to be tattooed on your forehead, so every time you look in the mirror you are reminded of what is going to be better when you take the leap in to health. I'm KIDDING! Getting really solid about what is not working and what life looks like now, because of your current habits, is critical.

Next, take that step to imagine what would change, if you change. I know it seems scary. But "new" is about action. So, as you start on this new lifestyle adventure. Before you slide back into an old habit, ask yourself one question: **Does this choice take me closer to my goal or further away.** If your answer is "further away, but, blah, blah, blah..." that is called an excuse - remember - a reason with a lie attached. That is your comfort zone kicking in. That is the comfy old way of thinking. Check yourself. Then make the uncomfy choice. For a while it will feel like a stone in your shoe, or a lump in your throat, or an ache in your heart.

Some of these thought patterns are so engrained they take months or years to change. So what? Barring a tragedy, you will be around for a long time. So, you might as well be healthy. This thought in and of itself may make you feel angry or sad or unmotivated. Or, it could make you feel giddy with anticipation.

So, let's talk about emotions for a bit. Jim Detmer in the 15 Habits of Conscious Leadership says that emotions are just "energy in motion". This energy will not kill you. This energy will create feelings. These feelings will not kill you. You may recognize them in certain parts of your body. Feel the feeling and name it, and where you feel it. Getting really clear that anger, sadness, fear, shame, joy or even sexual feelings are just feelings, they are just emotions. Just energy in motion. If we take the time to actually sit with the emotion, Detmer says it only lasts about 90 seconds. Okay, the emotion won't kill you and it only lasts 90 seconds. He also says you can process it if you name where you are feeling it, put a sound and some actual motion to it.

Now, I realize that when you get cut off in traffic the motions and sounds that you may make, um…may not be appropriate. So, you may have to find an appropriate place to finish processing certain emotions. Make sure you do it though. Then, you can manage and own your emotions instead of your emotions owning you. This will also allow you to see other people's emotions. You will not feel the need to "fix" everything. You will realize that they, too, need to learn how to manage their own emotions.

Being in charge of your feelings will help you stay in charge of your habits. Just because you 'feel" like having some ice cream, that may or may not be helping you toward your goal.

This is some of the new "hard" or "ridiculous" you face instead of looking at your current "stuck" life. This new hard is uncomfortable. My guess, so is looking at your current life. Really getting to the "why" of what I am changing has helped me get out of my own way and stop overthinking it. The things that I know are going to be SOO much better in my life are the things I stay focused on. I do not focus on the "hard" of making it happen. I feel the discomfort of the new habit. I reframe the feeling to mean excitement to grow, not nervousness about what people will think or that I can't do this because it's "just not me". It is going to be the "NEW" me! SOOOOO... which do you want, your current suckiness or a new awesomeness?

Now Actually Do It = ACTION!

Action is the difference between a dream and a goal. You can want something really bad, complain about it, start and stop for a million reasons, meditate on it, pray for it, wish for it, see yourself there, but until you take the first step, you are stuck in your day dreams.

Action is about application. Apply what you are learning.

What happens when you REALLY want something? Seriously, anything. Think about it, what did you last go out of your way to do or to get? Do you remember? Concert tickets to your favorite band? Something special for someone special? What about the time your big screen tv went out just a few days before the big game? A new top you saw on your favorite star? Some cool shoes you just had to have? Maybe something for your kids? Did you find the money for it? Did you find the time to do it? Did you let anything get in your way? How do those things compare to getting your health back? To losing the weight you want? To getting into shape? To really getting your life back?

This is the place where self-help books get a bad reputation. This is where "diets don't work" comes from... all of the BS in most of these books works if the advice is followed, even at 80-90%! Even this book. I have tons of evidence that these plans work when people work the plans.

When you get stuck ask yourself what is missing in your plan? Go back to the questions above. Remind yourself of where you started. Maybe you went to a birthday party, had some cake and didn't feel too bad, you unconsciously brought back sugar, slowly, in small quantities that over the past few weeks have grown into larger quantities. The holiday season that starts at the end of October through December is the most potent time for shifting back into negative habits.

Getting in the habit of asking yourself "what am I doing, is this (ACTION or DECISION) moving me closer to suckiness or awesomeness?" Closer to crapulous or fabulous? Then, start tracking your habits again. This will usually unearth the root of your "sudden" 5-pound weight gain, return of stomach issues, etc. We often underestimate the power of stressful events in our life. There is a mind-body connection. Events in our lives, even happy events like a graduation or a move, influence our health in ways that we don't always understand.

The key is to return to the positive habits. Ask, Act, Apply, Ask...rinse and repeat...

Where do you begin?

Start with the Current Realty Functional Health Check. It's on my website. Then, get into one of my online classes and start using the food plan I outlined in the Eat section of the Clean It Up chapter. Just start there. Work on getting yourself right with food. Food is fuel, nothing more. Just like emotions are energy in motion. If you need to lose weight and are frustrated, find me on Facebook, friend me and message me personally. I will let you know if you are a good fit for our plan. Just start with the basics. You can only control YOU! Eat, Drink, Move, Sleep Think and Feel.

Chapter 7: P: Personalized

It Really IS All About You

Personalized

P stands for many things. Personalized is first because it is at the core of the Functional Medicine philosophy. Functional Medicine has its roots in being a "Patient Centered" model. What that means is that instead of focusing on the disease, FM focuses on the patient who happens to have poor health. Yes, you may have a namable disease. You could have cancer, or auto-immune disorders, Irritable Bowel Syndrome, or just feel like CRAP! In any case you are a person first. We also believe the body can heal itself if it has all the right ingredients. Given the right nutrition and rest, the body innately knows what to do to be healthy. Maybe you have not set that up to happen in your body to this point in your life. Just know if it can happen for the thousands of people who have seen FM practitioners, it can happen for you too.

Creating a personalized plan is very important. You may be saying, but wait, you just wrote a book for the masses that said we should all do it your way. While that is true. There is a commonality amongst most of my patients over 25 years in practice. The fact that most "feel like CRAP" and have no energy says a lot. I believe that even those of you who have eaten clean most of your life can tweak something in your plan or may need a gentle reminder to shift back into good habits. Food is the easiest place to start.

Personalization will come in when you have cleaned up what you Eat, Drink, how you Move Sleep, Think and Feel. That is your foundation of health. Then, or at the same time, Clean up your gut. Digestion must be in order for your body to heal. You need those nutrients.

Personalized Testing

Personalized also means the plan is going to be somewhat unique for you. Before I launch into FM testing. All of the diagnostic tests your traditional doctor has done or suggests to do, need to be done. They will rule out all the ugly diagnoses. AND, even if you come up with some issue, the protocols you learn here will be beneficial and could heal you from the inside out. There are many tests FM doctors use to assess your personal health. I will talk about the ones I use, and feel are beneficial. This will differ by the doctor. We all have a little different perspective.

General Laboratory Testing

The following list is my Functional Health Panel. When you have labs done by your traditional doctor, you may have had some of these done and you were told "everything is fine". I have not seen one person with "Optimal Values". FM docs assess your labs with a different set of lab values. We call them "optimal values". These are the typical "healthy people" values.

From the FM perspective, we believe people start healthy and when stresses enter the system, your body will compensate for some time, then it will start falling apart. Most diseases are ones that accumulate over tie. Think about it. Heart disease doesn't happen overnight. The plaques didn't form in one evening. Diabetes, strokes, cancer, anemias, Vitamin D deficiencies, none of these conditions become apparent without a growth period. Your labs will reflect incremental changes over time. Traditional lab values are not designed to find those incremental changes. They find the problem when there is one. The "optimal values" allow us to find conditions before they become a real problem. Traditional doctors are taught to look for the disease, not the root. Traditional doctors are not trained to look at Optimal Values nor are they trained in nutrition as a form of treatment.

I will reiterate, traditionally trained doctors do a great job at treating acute, sudden illnesses or accidents. They are not really equipped to treat the lifestyle-based chronic disease epidemic in our country.

The following list of lab tests combine to tell a good chunk of the story about your health. I am going to give you some lab basics, so you can look at your own values from a different perspective. You can get into one of my online DIY-FM Lab classes from my website.

- ANA Screen, IFA, with Reflex to Titer and Pattern - a very general test that screens for over 250 autoimmune disorders. Just because it is positive, or you have a high titer, doesn't mean you are doomed. It just means you need to get your immune system under control.
- Ferritin - is considered the storage form of iron, but can be elevated during inflammation, and it is not always a good estimate of iron status
- Gamma Glutamyl Transferase (GGT) - glutathione, B6, magnesium status; traditionally elevated with excessive alcohol consumption.
- Hemoglobin A1c - Diabetes marker
- Magnesium - serum magnesium isn't always a good status marker for whether magnesium is actually inside your cells
- T3 Total - Active Thyroid hormone attached to protein plus free T3
- T3 Uptake - percent of freeT3 being taken up by the cell
- T4 Free - T4 available for conversion to T3. Conversion is nutrient dependent
- T4 (Thyroxine), Total - Thyroid hormone made by the thyroid, attached to thyroxine binding globulin protein
- T3, Free - Active thyroid hormone taken into the cell
- TSH - Thyroid stimulating hormone is from the pituitary, it is made in response to low T4 levels. When T4 drops, the pituitary produces TSH to stimulate the thyroid to make T4
- CBC (includes Differential and Platelets) - There are many markers in a CBC that tell us about iron and B12 status. HgB should be 13.5-14.5, clues about iron status; MCV - greater than 92 is telling about B12 status, if >92 = need for B12, and may be a clue to genetic factors influencing B-complex assimilation. if < 87 may mean low Iron, or the inability to assimilate iron.
- Thyroid Peroxidase and Thyroglobulin Antibodies - auto antibodies to the thyroid

- Iron, Total and Total Iron Binding Capacity - allows us to understand where the iron issue may be - root cause of iron deficiency
- Lipid Panel - cholesterol, triglycerides, HDL, LDL the body makes 75% of our cholesterol. Cholesterol is necessary for normal hormone production. It is NOT necessarily the only cause of heart disease. We need lipids to make healthy cell membranes. The healthy membranes of each cell allow appropriate communication from cell to cell.
- hs-CRP - an inflammatory marker, primarily indicating cardiovascular disease, stroke and diabetes
- Comprehensive Metabolic Panel - gives us an idea about kidney, liver, electrolyte function, pH, adrenals, protein status
- Vitamin D, 25-Hydroxy, Total, Immunoassay - vitamin D is a primary player to decrease inflammation, keep the immune system under control, is necessary for healthy bones and brain function.
- Homocysteine - is an inflammatory molecule that gives us a clue about our B6, folate and B12 status.

Food Sensitivity Testing

Let's be clear here...we really need to be really clear about terminology. This is not the same as allergy testing. Allergy testing is testing for Immunoglobulin E, or IgE, immediate reaction to a food, environmental substances, or chemicals. These are immediate reactions that can cause death! Most adults are aware of foods that cause these immediate reactions. The food sensitivity testing is not generally accepted by traditional doctors. Having a delayed reaction, in their eyes is not life threatening therefore may or may not be clinically relevant. After testing thousands of patients over 25 years, I have found that when patients identify what they are sensitive to, and remove it for at least 90 days, many symptoms like headaches, IBS, stomach pain, acne, joint pain, low energy and others go away! You also may be more motivated to stay away from gluten and dairy when you see that your body is reacting negatively to it...

If you have had a leaky gut, you may find you have many low-level food sensitivities. It may be an indicator of "leakiness".

Adrenal Hormone Testing

This is a salivary test. Usually 4 samples are taken throughout the day. This will tell us how your adrenals are functioning and if you have a normal cortisol rhythm. Cortisol levels should be higher in the morning and decrease through the day. This allows you to wake up ready to face the day, and ready to go to sleep naturally in the evening. When you have been adrenally fatigued for an extended period of time, the cortisol levels can be flat through the day or go up in the evening. There are many patterns that can result. This test really requires a professional to interpret. Your traditionally trained doctor is not educated in salivary testing. If you have followed the steps through this book and you are still having a fatigue, this may be a good test for you to discover the root cause of your fatigue.

Stool Testing/Comprehensive Digestive Analysis

This is different testing than what your traditional doctor will offer you. A good stool test will take 3 different samples over the course of a week or so. It will identify the type of bacteria and if there are any pathogenic ("Bad") bacteria. It should also tell the doctor what natural herbs will actually kill the bad dudes.

Figuring out the root causes may require some additional testing. I typically start with my Functional Health Panel and the Food Sensitivity testing. Because I really want this book to be a DIY book, starting with Eat, Drink, Move Sleep Think and Feel; then following through the Gut Healing, Liver Detoxification and Regeneration, along with the Hormone/Adrenal Rebuild plan will put you in a much healthier place. Then, you can use the testing to tweak your plan to be a little more personalized.

The Plan

You will need a Plan. Our Current Reality Functional Health Check is the perfect place to start. Get your score and start one of my online classes. I created these online classes, so you could start fixing your health in a meaningful way without having to search and search the internet, and NOT have a clue where to start.

Start eating what I outlined in the EAT chapter. It's a place to start. This healing thing is a journey. It's a trip. We are going to start in one place and end up somewhere else. The somewhere else will be there. Exactly how healthy you will be in the future depends on what you are willing to do today, and the next day and next week and next month for the next six months to a year. Then, next year at this time, take a pause, look at what you have done for yourself.

The thing about traveling is there are sometimes unexpected things that crop up. As I finish writing this book, I am sitting at LAX because I just missed a flight. Oh well, life happens, and the hiccup on this journey is giving me 3 more hours than I would have had if I just went home on my previously scheduled flight.

When things happen on our trek, it has nothing to do with the "thing" and everything to do with how we chose to respond to it. Sure, was I upset? Yep, for a bit, then I settled in and realized I had a better chance of actually finishing my book because of the delay.

People

People will be people. Their reaction to what you are doing has nothing to do with you! This is a valuable lesson as you move forward in your healing journey. You chose how you respond to them. If you have used food as your escape hatch for your entire life, you may actually believe it is "just the way you are" but that doesn't have to be "who you are" forever.

Does starting this program mean you have to give up your favorite foods for the rest of your life? NO! It does mean that you need to give your body a chance to heal. Going gluten free for a week then allowing yourself birthday cake at your kid's party is not okay this year. Yes, this is with the most love and grace and hugs and support I can muster. The exceptions have to actually be exceptions, not the rule every weekend.

"But I will hurt people's feelings." I hear this all the time. Here's the thing. People in your life may or may not agree with what you have chosen to do for yourself. Some may be scared, others down right offended, others passive aggressive and trying to sabotage you, that is their emotion. Your choices may offend people. It is still YOUR choice for YOUR life. When we take a stand, people get upset. They don't understand how it might effect them. They get angry, sad, jealous, upset, pissy, scared, or any number of other negative responses. THAT'S OKAY! That is <u>their</u> response and as nothing to do with YOU! It is <u>THEIR</u> response. The sooner we learn to let people emote, realize it's not our emotion to manage, and love them anyway, the sooner we can on with empowering ourselves to a better place. Allow yourself to make new supportive friends. Find our online support group on Facebook. We created for you! Get into one of my online classes and you will find kindred spirits traversing the same trail.

Perfectionism

This brings me to the next "P". Perfectionism. Perfectionism will not be tolerated! I say that with lots of love and grace, as a recovering perfectionist. This book had 3 false starts because of fear. I was afraid you wouldn't like it, people wouldn't like me, it wouldn't be good enough, I would have nothing of value to say, and many other negative self-esteem BS chit-chats with myself.

How much of that BS runs in your head?

This fear is part of a self-limiting belief system that has its roots in shame. We went through some Limiting Belief Basics earlier in the book. I can speak from personal experience but if you really want the expert on shame and perfectionism, I believe Brene Brown is awesome! Her work changed my life and is partially responsible for me moving forward with this project. Go to the additional resources on my website.

I also want to bring up perfectionism because many of us struggle with trying to be everything to everyone. That generally means we are actually nothing to no one. You are going to let people down, you cannot live up to others' expectations all the time. It's part of being human. Don Miguel Ruiz wrote a book called The Four Agreements. It helps to do my best to remember these:

1. Be impeccable with your word. Do your best to follow through on doing what you say you are going to do. We not only let the other person down when we don't, we also erode trust in ourselves. Honor your commitments. Use words in love not harm. Blame and criticism do little to actually improve relationships. Take responsibility for your actions and your words.

2. Don't take anything personally. We can choose to take the opinions of others as truth or NOT! People choose their own actions. No one does anything BECAUSE of someone. They may respond, they may blame but it is still their choice what they do with their words and actions. Ruiz puts it this way: "Nothing other people do is because of you."

3. Don't make assumptions. Seriously, we are all guilty and do it so automatically we don't even realize it. The problem is, we believe them to be truth! When we believe falsehoods to be true, we take it personally, and it creates a vicious circle. Until you have clarified it with that person, or group, you are making assumptions. Stop the negative chit-chat in your head...or at least start paying attention to it. Ask lots of questions until you clarify the situation. Clarification rocks!

4. Always do you best. NOT PERFECT! Some days you are a Rock Star and some days you are a slug... kidding, but right? You know when you are doing your best, even on your bad days. This is not about "should", a different conversation. When you are not doing your best, depression, and anxiety bubble up. The idea here is to beseeching improvement all the time. What is a fail today, is the lesson of tomorrow.

Shoulda, Woulda, Coulda.

Listen to how many times you say, "I should have done XY or Z." Or "I would have done X if …" Or "I could have done that if…" These are the root of many self-limiting beliefs and guilt. They also place you firmly in the past. When we live in the past, depression reigns. Get this now, what can be changed about the past? NOTHING! Fails happen. Life happens, we are human. Forgiveness of the past and ourselves is crucial to healing. Take this journey with a counselor, Pastor, Rabi, or trusted, objective friend who speaks truth into you and will call you out gently when you need it. Forgiveness is key. Let it go. Nothing you can really change except how you respond to similar situations in the future.

Quick note about forgiveness. It is for YOU. It does not excuse the other persons actions. It does not stop consequences to the other person. What forgiveness does do is it releases that person from continuing to have a strongly on you. Chances are when someone wrongs you, they have forgotten all about it. But, you holding onto it keeps them in your life. Why would you want to keep holding onto a person or event that hurt you? What good is that doing? It's like you drinking the poison and expecting it to hurt the other person. Forgive them and move on!

So, ask yourself: "What can I learn and do differently NOW?"

The answer will propel you forward into action. Maybe you have stopped and started more health journeys than you can count. You have lost trust in yourself. Now you have a coach and a guide. This book, the online class, videos and forums to keep you accountable. You can make the changes you want to make. I know it feels weird and hard. And as I started this chapter, which do you want? Crapulous or Fabulous? Your current suckiness or new awesomeness?

Try this. For one week, sleep on the other side of the bed. Get up with a different alarm and eat something different for breakfast. Everything looks different, right?? Try getting up 30 minutes earlier to move your body. Even if you put your headphones on and dance in your living room. Everything feels so weird! That is what change feels like. You will want to slip back to your comfy old ways, but try embracing the excitement of the new and daring adventure you are beginning.

Peace in the Process

All of this is a process. You must take care of yourself. There is NOTHING selfish about eating healthy when your family chooses CRAP, there is nothing wrong with going to bed early because you are tired. There is nothing wrong with saying NO when you need to say NO. People have to learn to deal with their own emotions, just like you are learning to deal with yours, as I said earlier.

Working through all the years you have spent fighting with your health is a Process. To really go deeper into how you got sick, there are a couple options. The first module of my online class walks you through some pretty tough questions to help you discover the root causes and your timeline. Once you realize your past habits arrive created where your health is today, it can be changed. You can take charge of your habits and your health.

CRAP is a whole process. It is designed to keep you on your path. AND to pick you up when you have fallen off the wagon. You CAN keep doing this for life. It gets easier with time.

The sequence of CRAP is to clean it up. Figure out what needs to be cleaned up. From your diet to a closet or the basement, this process will work. Restore Function next. You may have to have some special nutrition, or if it's the closet, maybe some shelves, or paint. Action, without action, everything stays the same. Crapulous or Fabulous? Current suckiness or new awesomeness? Personalize it, lifestyle changes or closets need to be the way YOU want it.

Having this as a process to get yourself back on track is valuable. You never have to be far away from health. If you get off the track, fall off the wagon, just apply CRAP. First of all, it's kind of funny to think about going off the track via eating CRAP can lead you back to CRAP. (Yes, I know, I'm a dork to laugh at my own stuff.)

Clean it up, Restore function, Act on it, Personalize it.

CRAP is your safety net. You do not have to stay in the fail. You do not have to be a victim of your own choices. Go back to CRAP! And laugh, it's good medicine.

It takes perseverance, with a lot of self-love and grace. I have seen thousands go from Crapulous to Fabulous! You totally got this CRAP! CRAP!

Conclusion

We started our journey together by working on your health. When you open your mind, and get out of your own way, great things start happening in your life.

Our goal was to help you get your health back to Optimal and make sure you have the energy to live the life you deserve. To accomplish this, you must understand your exactly where you are, even if it is yucky right now because you feel like C.R.A.P!
Don't wait till you have it all together, there is never a good time.

Making sure you find someone that will guide you through the process is the fastest and best way to get your health back. If I haven't said it enough, you need a coach! Contact me or get my online course to walk you through it.

Once you understand and implement what you have learned in this book, you are on your way to your best health ever.

Don't forget to get your bonus at **bonus.Drkrissargent.com** as I put together information that will give you a clear picture on the how you can live the life you desire and deserve.

Congratulations!

It is time to first celebrate your victory. You created a goal of finishing this book, and now you have accomplished it. It is very important to take time, even if it can only be a moment, to celebrate your victories.

Recognize that you are one step closer to reaching your goal. Know that we are proud of your success and very grateful that you took the time to learn and consider how you are going to implement our teachings.

Your next step is to nurture these lessons and then take massive action!

"Inaction breeds doubt and fear. Action breeds confidence and courage. If you want to conquer fear, do not sit home and think about it. Go out and get busy"

~ Dale Carnegie

To your health!!!